THINK FIT 2 BE FIT

THINK FIT 2 BE FIT

A WEIGHT LOSS PROGRAM FOR
THE HEART, SOUL, BODY & MIND

TAMMY POLENZ

TATE PUBLISHING & Enterprises

Published by Tate Publishing & Enterprises, LLC
127 E. Trade Center Terrace | Mustang, Oklahoma 73064 USA
1.888.361.9473 | www.tatepublishing.com

Tate Publishing is committed to excellence in the publishing industry. The company reflects the philosophy established by the founders, based on Psalm 68:11,
"The Lord gave the word and great was the company of those who published it."

Book design copyright © 2011 by Tate Publishing, LLC. All rights reserved.
Cover design by Kellie Southerland
Interior design by Lindsay B. Behrens
Photographs by Tammy Mellert
Graphics by Harnett Chidede-Shimelonis
Logo design by Julia Briggs

Published in the United States of America

ISBN: 978-1-61739-384-6
1. Health & Fitness / Weight Loss   2. Health & Fitness / Healthy Living
11.01.17

Dedication

God
My foundation and the one responsible for every bless-
ing in my life. Thank you for always being there for me!

Nathan and Anthony
My sons, the source of my inspiration to be
the best I can be and to never give up!

Rusty Fischer
The man that helped me finish what I started.

Jim Breen
Thank you for standing by your every word.

Clients, Members, and Friends
Thank you to everyone over the many years that
have shared a part of their lives with me and
allowed me to share my passion with them.

My Team
Thank you for working with me to bring my dream
to fruition. Your work ethic, support, and passion
makes every day a treasured gift working with you.

Table of Contents

Introduction

Let's face it: we all know the statistics about obesity in adults and children, in poor people and rich people, in city people and rural folks. According to the National Health and Nutrition Examination Survey, for instance, nearly *two-thirds of adults in the United States are overweight* (meaning an individual is carrying more weight than is prescribed by certain national standards), and almost *one-third of those Americans that are overweight can be classified as obese* (a term that refers to an abnormally high proportion of body fat).

But it's one thing to hear the numbers and quite another to literally face the facts. So let's create a mental picture to bring these statistics to life. Let's say you are sitting in a room with twelve random strangers. Well, according to these national statistics, an amazing eight of them would be overweight—and four would be obese. That means, out of twelve modern Americans, only four would be considered "normal" weight.

For the first time in history, those considered to weigh a "normal" weight (according to national standards) aren't just outnumbered by the overweight and obese, but they are quickly becoming the exception versus the norm. In short, there are more overweight people in this country than there are "normal" weight people.

Why, according to CNN.com/Health, do we weigh four times more now than we did back in the 1980s? The surgeon general states that there are three main causes behind overweight and obesity:

(1) Lack of physical exercise
(2) Poor nutrition
(3) Poor health literacy

The solution seems obvious: if you *exercise, eat right,* and *educate yourself,* not only will you lose weight, but you will also be proactively involved in the prevention of disease in your own lifetime. The important thing to understand here is that the real problem is not that America is overweight.

Instead, America's weight issue is just a symptom of a much deeper problem. The *real* problem evidenced by these startling statistics is that we live in a society consisting of sedentary, poorly-nourished individuals who, despite all the information out there on how to eat and move right, are still uneducated about what it takes to be fit and healthy. What's amazing is that these national statistics seem at odds with a country that is so smart, so wealthy, so motivated, so proud, and so accomplished in so many other areas of life.

We can put men and women on the moon, create computers that work at the speed of light, write staggering works of genius, create billion-dollar summer blockbusters, cure diseases, feed the homeless, and create great symphonies—then listen to them on iPods smaller than most credit cards—yet we just can't figure out how to lose those last fifteen or twenty pounds!

How can this be? The simple fact is that we are not overweight because we don't think about it enough. After all, talk to any one person for any length of time, let alone a whole group of people, and before long the conversation will always come back to weight. Who's too fat, who's too skinny, who's on a diet, who's just fallen off of one—we are a nation obsessed with being overweight, and yet we are a nation that is literally more overweight than under.

No, the problem isn't how *much* we think about being overweight; it's *how* we think about being overweight. In short, the reason you are reading this book isn't because of how much you eat or how little you move; it's because of *how you think.*

If you think you can lose weight, you will.

If you think you can't, you won't.

Our problem is that we don't think we can really accomplish our goals; we don't believe that we can stick to our program, our routine, our diet, our gym membership, our resolution, or our commitment to simply lose weight.

We have failed so many times that we just can't honestly believe we can succeed this time. And we're partly right; we can't succeed if we don't think we can succeed.

The challenge with sticking to most programs, diets, gyms, or even diet books out there is that they leave the thinking out completely. By focusing on the body alone—on fat and protein, calories and grams, trans fats and carbs, etc.—those other programs ignore the very real, sophisticated, challenging, enlightening way in which how we think about what we do affects the outcome.

Yes, too many calories and not enough exercise add up to excess weight; that is a physical, scientific, and quantifiable fact without dispute. However, facts alone do not tell the whole story. How we think about the food we eat, how we work out, and even when, where, and why all go into how many calories we feel comfortable taking in without working them off.

The fact is we are not simply machines, consuming calories and expending them like a car takes in gas and shoots out motion. We are challenging, complex, and creative individuals, and we get emotional about our food. We eat when we're nervous, scared, happy, sad, or just simply bored. Animals don't have "comfort foods" like meat loaf, mashed potatoes, macaroni and cheese, and pumpkin pie; they eat what they can scavenge and are happy for it!

We are the only creatures on the planet that put so much thought, effort, work, and joy into not just what we eat but how we eat it, when, and where. We have cooking shows, gourmet restaurants, best-selling cookbook authors, celebrity chefs, and entire streets of our cities and towns devoted to food, food, and more food.

If food is so central to our thought process, how can we leave the thought process out of eating less food? The answer is simple: we can't. So my new book, *Think Fit 2 Be Fit: A Weight Loss Program for the Heart, Soul, Body, and Mind,* doesn't leave out the thought process; in fact, it creates an entirely *new* thought process so you can finally believe that success is attainable.

Who am I, and why should you listen to my philosophy about weight loss? My name is Tammy Polenz, and as a single mom of two boys, business owner, and avid athlete that has competed in fitness shows on a national level, I truly understand how the hectic pace of life can leave little time for personal wellness. I also recognize the unique challenges that a modern childhood can bring to those seeking healthful decisions in a sea of fast, quick, and junk offerings.

Like many young women growing up, I went through a dreadful time regarding my weight. I endured severe low self-esteem and poor self-image in my early teenage years and would starve myself for extended periods of time, which was followed by bouts of eating binges that might last for days or even weeks. My weight would fluctuate by as much as twenty pounds within as little as thirty days. Even when weighing as little as 102 pounds, I was still not satisfied with the way I looked or felt physically.

At the age of sixteen, while randomly flipping through TV channels one day, I came across a show on ESPN hosted by Corey Everson called *Body Shaping.* Corey and her team were promoting fitness via weight training. Both the men and women on the show looked incredible and possessed the most athletic bodies I had ever seen. At that moment, I immediately knew that this was what I had been trying to achieve the entire time. Not only was Corey's show promoting toned physiques, but they also discussed the importance of overall health and well-being by consuming a balanced diet.

My life changed from that moment forward because it was the first time in my young life that I was able to make the connection between having a fit physique and overall wellness. This was when my journey into fitness began, during which time I implemented the information I was learning to create proactive habits that would lead me toward reaching my goal of obtaining the fit body I so desperately desired. Along the way, the changes in my overall health and vitality for the better were what finally sold me on the concept of living a fit lifestyle. And after my life changed so drastically, well, I couldn't help but pass along what I had learned to others.

While working as a personal fitness trainer and wellness coach over the last twenty years, I have gained extensive knowledge and experience in the areas of nutrition, post-rehabilitation, resistance training, weight management, sports-specific conditioning, and more. I take immense pleasure in working with people of all ages and abilities, and I have instructed hundreds of clients, both in a one-on-one environment as well as group settings, assisting them in reaching their uniquely personalized health and wellness goals.

Now it's your turn! I truly believe that *Think Fit 2 Be Fit* is *the* program that is going to help you change your life, much the same way a simple TV program changed mine. We all need to start somewhere, and for me, the mind is the best place to start.

So let's not waste another moment, shall we?

Let's learn what it really means to *Think Fit 2 Be Fit!*

STEP 1:

Think Fit 2 Be Fit

Throughout my childhood and most of my teenage years, I really had no concept of serving sizes. When my step-dad would cook French toast for breakfast, for instance (which, by the way, was my favorite breakfast food), I would eat half a loaf of it myself. Then, to top it off, I'd pile loads of powdered sugar on it.

Corn on the cob was another favorite treat of mine. When my mom would buy it during its prime harvest season, she'd buy twelve ears for the family and twelve ears just for me! And let me tell you, I'd eat every one of those twelve ears in one sitting, smothered in butter and covered in salt too. Yum, talk about overeating!

It's amazing to think I could have eaten that much by myself—and that was *before* I started having weight problems. I guess that's how people get started on bad habits and find it difficult to change once they find them-selves in their adult years. See, when we were kids, many

Believing you can means eliminating all negative thoughts. Negative thoughts create mental blocks and prevent you from focusing on the positive changes that get results. An example of one such block is realizing that getting in shape and losing weight is a lifestyle, not an event.

That's key to the *Think Fit 2 Be Fit* mentality: this won't happen all overnight; these are habits you build up over time. Remember, you didn't gain all that weight or get out of shape in a day, right? So losing the weight and getting in shape will—and should—take time as well. Having a positive outlook about health and fitness will make walking the path of success effortless and speedy.

Believing you can do something entails a shift change in your thinking, and to make that shift you will need to do a few things to start the process.

Part of the *Think Fit 2 Be Fit* mentality starts with flooding your mind with proactive information, like what you will find here, that will teach you more about yourself and how to get where you want to be. When you flood your brain with information, an incredible thing happens. The information will begin to change your belief system. As your beliefs change, your actions will follow. The more you do something, the easier it becomes, and the more apt you are to continue doing it until those actions eventually become consistent habits.

The more you do something, the higher the probability it will create change. Changes both positive and negative reinforce behavior. If seeing is believing and doing equates to outcomes that you can see, then the actions you change will reinforce the belief and confidence you have in yourself.

THOUGHT TO FRUITION

What is the difference between an Olympic athlete and you? Just one thing: your frame of mind! That's right: *fitness is nothing more than a mind-set.* Specifically, it is a set of beliefs that you hold about yourself. Those beliefs paint a picture of who are to yourself and to the world around you. They determine what you are capable of accomplishing before you even try. Of course, genetics plays a role to some degree, but the most important component in reaching any goal depends on two basic points:

(1) Your mental focus and...
(2) The way you view yourself.

Look at your computer, for instance. It needs to be programmed to work, and so does your brain. Think of it another way: there is a little person upstairs in that head of yours taking notes all day and all night while you are sleeping, awake, eating, watching TV, showering, daydreaming, working, not listening to someone even though you're supposed to be, or whatever you might be doing. Your brain is always recording everything that is happening around you. What is he or she taking notes about? Everything! Everything you have seen, heard, and felt, both physically and emotionally. This includes what others say to you, what you say aloud, your internal dialogue, what you see with your eyes, what you visualize mentally, and any other sensations you might pick up on throughout the day.

The important thing to realize regarding your brain is that every single inputted message, energetic sensation, or thought that occurs is permanently stored into your memory at some level. Whether you consciously remember or not, it is there. Under hypnotism, people remember some of the most intricate details about an incident, like what color shirt a person was wearing, the smell of their perfume, a license plate number, or whether the water was dripping in the background or not.

The information your brain collects can be stored in short-term or long-term memory. Short-term memory covers periods from a fraction of a second to a few minutes or more, whereas long-term memory covers hours, days, months, or even years. Through repetition, or when strong emotions are evoked, short-term memory can become long-term memory. At any level, your brain thinks all incoming information is factual and true until otherwise proven different.

Knowing how the brain works is a crucial component for creating a fit body, because *you are what your mind thinks you are.* "What the mind conceives, the body achieves," it is said, not the other way around. Your thoughts create the person you are today. The great news for your health and fitness is that those beliefs about who you are and what you can achieve are not set in stone. Your brain is plastic in nature and can be remolded to believe something very different from what you believe today. For instance, if you believe you are unhealthy and unable to attain a fit and healthy body, you can retrain your brain to believe that you are a fit, lean, tone, positive-orientated, healthy person. If you were to believe you were all these things and more, how do you think you might live your life differently?

REPETITION, THE MOTHER
OF RETENTION

Motivation is what gives you the drive to participate in a new exercise program or eating plan. The problem occurs when that initial fire that got you started burns out and you do not yet possess the constructive habits that will keep you moving toward your goals. What is the secret to retaining your motivation over time?

One thing: habitual behavior, or, as they're more frequently called, "habits."

MSN Encarta defines a habit as "a regularly repeated behavior pattern: an action or pattern of behavior that is repeated so often that it becomes typical of somebody, although he or she may be unaware of it."

Habits are reflex behaviors; eventually they become an involuntary action you just do without even thinking about it anymore. Take, for instance, the habit of brushing your teeth. Everybody does it, or at least we hope they do. When you were young, your parents may have had to remind you repeatedly to brush your teeth, or what is better stated "programmed" you to brush your teeth. Through repetition, the once seemingly annoying chore has become an ingrained habit over time. It was hard to remember at first, but now you do not even think about it; you just do it.

Through time and the creation of hundreds of habits, you have created what is now your present lifestyle. Good or bad, your lifestyle is nothing more than a set of behaviors that you or someone else trained you to do. These habitual behaviors either produce desired living conditions or undesirable ones.

One example of how your thoughts and behaviors can change subconsciously is when you start hanging out with a new friend. That little person is up in your head taking notes, even if you are unaware that it is going on. The next thing you know, you are using words your new friend often uses and practicing habits they have, good or bad. Why does this happen? Audio and visual repetition is the culprit.

Due to hearing the same words repeatedly and seeing or participating in repetitive behaviors, you begin to pick them up and incorporate them into your own lifestyle without even realizing it. This is the same principle children use in learning how to walk and talk; it is a psychological function called mirroring.

Children watch and listen to their parents and the people around them, taking notes of everything around them, just like you do when learning something new. The next thing you know they are little mirrors of their parents by walking, talking, and acting just like them. This is our natural way of learning and precisely why children learn from what they see and not by what they are told. Adults are all just little children on the inside, learning and becoming who they are through sensory experience.

Advertisers use repetition in marketing as a way to make consumers more comfortable with buying their products. After seeing a product advertised hundreds of times, the majority of people will feel more comfortable buying it. In fact, this tactic works so well that people will never forget their products.

Morgan Spurlock's revolutionary *Super Size Me* is one of the best fast-food documentaries on the market today. It depicts how strongly people are influenced by these advertising moguls. In one segment of the documentary, children were asked to identify some pictures of historical characters. When asked to identify a picture of George Washington, they did very poorly. When asked to identify pictures of Jesus, none of the children in the documentary were able to tell Morgan who he was. Lastly, when asked to identify Ronald McDonald, each and every one of the children knew exactly who this character was, without hesitation.

It is mind-boggling to see the effects of market programming and its effects on our psyche in live action. You and I are no different than these children. We are programmed just as easily, and programming changes our thoughts, which drives all of our decisions, good and bad.

Another way you store memories, which lead to the beliefs you own and actions you take, is when emotions are involved. When strong emotions are ignited, memories are more easily stored, and, therefore, habits are more easily created.

Here is an example that might resonate with you. As a young boy, Tommy watches his father building a doghouse. The father is lost in the project at hand and hammering away, when all of a sudden, instead of hitting the nail, he hits his own finger. His first reaction is to yell, "Damn!" This, of course, causes a strong, emotional response in the boy, because his father got hurt and it startled little Tommy at the same time.

This strong, emotional response by the child allows this particular moment to be stored in his long-term memory. The effect? Every time little Tommy hurts himself, he yells, "Damn!" Not an uncommon story, right? The problem now is breaking the child of this action or new habit he has developed, a poor habit created by an intense emotional response. The point is that repetition and strong emotions cause habits to be stored in long-term memory and, therefore, are hard to change or break.

A poor habit many people suffer from is emotional eating, which is created in relation to strong, emotional responses. At some point in time, emotional distress followed by eating gave the person suffering from emotional eating problems a sense of ease or release, so they continued this negative eating pattern long after the first time. The foods associated with emotional eating are usually junk or comfort foods because of their physiological response in the body, which is similar to that of drugs.

Here is a great way to see a poor habit spring to life. First, we have a cause, emotional distress. Next is the effect or action that some individuals take, which is to eat in response to the emotional distress. The secondary problem, other than eating for the wrong reasons, is that most individuals that take part in emotional eating usually go for high calorie junk food choices. Highly processed foods with loads of sugar cause a drug-like effect. Sugar causes your body to release serotonin, a feel-good hormone, which produces a sense of calm afterward.

Repeat this process time after time, for weeks, months, or even years, and you have a habit so ingrained it is seemingly impossible to change. This type of habit is a little tougher to change because it is caused by a strong, emotional response and repetition and then locked in via a drug-like response by the body. Though this type of habit is difficult to break, it is not impossible.

FOLLOW THE LEADER

Well, now that you know what causes bad habits, how do you change them or build new, positive ones? If you don't like your current situation, then you need to start changing it by changing your habits. To create new habits, you need to repeat an action or behavior over and over again. Then through repetition of new, proactive behaviors, you will produce new habits and the lifestyle you desire, along with its outcome. These new habits paint the picture of life exactly the way your heart desires it to be. All it takes is some work and focus.

There is no magic pill, secret potion, or guarantee: people who are fit *live* fit; it's just that simple. It's a daily, ongoing process that frankly never stops. The good news is that once you *are* fit, you really don't want it to stop. Simply going through the motions and doing what healthy people do is the best way to get started creating new habits.

One of the simple, standard, and regular things fit people do is set goals and achieve them. In the next step, we will talk more specifically about goals and how to reach them, but for now, just know this: goals are the cornerstone for every weight loss and fitness success.

So, for a moment, pretend that you have already reached your fitness goals. If you already attained your goals today, how do you suppose your lifestyle would be different? What would be different about it specifically? What choices would you make on a daily basis, and/or what behaviors would you stay away from?

One example of how someone would act differently if they were already fit that I have heard over the years is when someone tells me that they would start going to the gym once they lost some weight. What? That does not even make sense. Why not go to the gym to lose weight in the first place? This is a perfect example of how you can apply the action now, as though you have already attained your goal. They say it takes eighteen to twenty-one days to create a new habit, so between now and then, practice productive actions each day until it becomes so ingrained that it is an involuntary action.

If you really want to get fit, do what a fit person does. Find an athlete and ask what they do. Study them, just as you would study any other subject you want to learn about. When you want to excel in something, you study every aspect of it and then implement what you learn. There are athletes all around you, such as personal train-ers (as long as they practice what they preach), kids in sports, the friend everyone refers to as the "health nut," or you can just read about fit people in magazines. As you research, pay attention to what they eat and eat the same things. Ask them how many days they work out a week and for how long and then do that. Remember, a true athlete or fit person does not work for a couple of weeks or a couple of months or even a year before they get in shape. A true athlete or fit individual lives a healthy lifestyle every day, every month, every year for their entire life. This is what you need to do—live a healthy lifestyle for the rest of your life. Then and only then will you never have to worry about your weight again.

I know you may not have goals of becoming an Olympic athlete, and I am not saying that you need to, especially if your goal is to just get in shape. What I am saying to do is adopt a fitness frame of mind, and your actions and body will follow. Getting fit means getting healthy from the inside out. As mentioned before, "What the mind conceives the body achieves," not the other way around. So produce something better by conceiving something better.

HEALTH LITERACY

The surgeon general states that the three major causes of overweight and obesity are (1) lack of physical activity, (2) poor nutrition, and (3) poor health literacy. According to the Harvard School of Public Health, Department of Society, Human Development and Health, health literacy is "the degree to which individuals have the capacity to obtain, process, and understand basic health information and services needed to make appropriate health decisions." In other words, taking what you have learned and applying it to your life. But what if the info you have is wrong? It is imperative that you be able to identify accurate information. False information is all around us. It's in the media, newspapers, magazines, on TV, the radio, just about everywhere, because of marketing gimmicks of companies trying to make money off of the uneducated consumer. I've seen weight loss and/or fitness advertisements in magazines these days that encompass a several page spread, which depicts graphs and charts demonstrating high success rates and biased studies to support the sale of their products. To the consumer, the product looks legitimate and may even work to cause some weight loss, but it is just another quick fix and will not last. Many products over the years have even led to hospitalization from adverse reactions.

The key is to find reliable studies and information that are nonbiased and provided by credible resources, such as health professionals, certified fitness coaches, or associations like the American Diabetic Association, the American Heart Association, the American Dietetic Association, and the Center for Disease Control and Prevention, or CDC. These sources will provide you with accurate, reliable, and safe information that will enable you to reach your weight-management goals through healthy consumer decisions.

As mentioned earlier, by saturating your brain with fitness-focused, accurate information, you will be encouraged to make proactive decisions. Therefore, look for and absorb information related to healthy lifestyle, well-balanced nutrition, healthy meal preparation, proper exercise, injury prevention, holistic health, and any other health-related topics that will aid you in your efforts toward attaining your personal fitness goals.

ATTENTION TO FITNESS

Remember learning about selective attention in junior high? It is when you orient yourself toward something or focus your attention and awareness toward one part of your environment but exclude other parts. This is the same process that happens when you buy a new car and then drive it down the street, suddenly noticing every other car of the same make and model as yours. You may do the same with clothing, paint colors, furniture, sports, or even food.

A perfect example of this is when you keep telling yourself that you cannot have any chocolate because you are on a diet. The problem is that suddenly, thanks to selective attention, the only thing you think about is chocolate! Well, that's like saying, "Do not think of pink elephants." What happens? You picture a pink elephant in your mind almost immediately, and it is just about impossible not to think about them, even though you are trying not to.

Whatever you tell yourself to stop thinking about or try to avoid in your life, like chocolate, is exactly where your mind is going to wander. Whatever is on your mind is going to drive your actions. Ever wonder why you crave chocolate or your favorite junk food more after you have told yourself that you cannot have it? Now you know: selective attention.

The key to success is to keep your attention focused on the things that will create proactive behaviors and drive positive choices. If your goal is to eat healthier and consume less junk food, instead of thinking about all the things you cannot have, think about all the things you *can* have. This keeps your brain focused on thoughts that will drive positive actions, instead of negative ones. Remember our discussion on positive habitual behavior? Successful people do this regularly; focusing on the positive is a habit for them.

One example of where I use selective attention is when dining out. Most individuals that are trying to make healthier choices in their diets will typically scan a menu and find all the things they cannot have, like dessert. I have created the habit of looking for only those items that will help me reach my goals. Therefore, when searching a menu for meal options, I will look at the salad selection or non-pasta dishes. Grilled and baked selections that are high protein choices are tops on my list, along with choices that are not drenched in sauces or butter.

I also frequent restaurants that are open to exchanging food items that come with an entree, such as vegetables in place of starches for those evening meals. Be sure to remain focused on those foods, choices, behaviors, and actions that will get you the outcome you desire.

For instance, when grocery shopping, choose to walk the store perimeter first, filling your cart with healthier food items. If you think about it, the outer perimeter of the store aisles is where the fresh produce, meat, fish, poultry, and one-ingredient foods are stocked, whereas the inner aisles are where are the highly processed foods are shelved. Use selective attention to direct you toward places where the healthiest choices are easily found. Farmers' markets during various seasons are great locations to find whole foods as well.

THINK YOURSELF THIN

Your brain is the single most important tool that you can use to accomplish anything you want in life. The power of thought is how everything around you has come into existence. Think about it. What was once science fiction is now reality: cell phones, skyscrapers, airplanes, and traveling into outer space. Every possibility starts with a thought and is then brought into existence via focus, determination, and effort through action. There are several studies, books, and other pieces of literature that provide support to the concept of "mind over matter."

In fact, did you know that the very act of thinking literally changes the shape of the brain? Brain cells that fire together link together, so the more actions, thoughts, and feelings that your brain is involved with every day, the more brain cells that will fire and link up together. If you want your actions to change, you have to change your thoughts first, which will therefore cause different cells to fire, literally changing the shape of your brain and eventually locking those actions into permanent behaviors.

This is precisely why habits get so ingrained into a person's lifestyle; people actually do get stuck in a rut. A more accurate description of what occurs is that brain cells clump together via firing, which keeps a person stuck in those patterns of behavior and thought, good or bad.

Not only will thinking change the shape of your brain, but it can also change your body's chemistry and physical appearance. Think about it: do you walk taller when you are happy? Do you walk more slumped over and slower when you are sad? These are just two examples of how your thoughts can affect your body structure.

If you are chronically sad, your body posture will adjust and conform in an alignment that reflects this. What about physiology? If I tell you to think about taking a bite into a sour lemon, it will probably make your mouth pucker due to its sour and tart mouth-watering juices. What happens? Does your mouth start watering as though you have that lemon right in front of you? Of course it does; this is one physiological change that you notice simply from your thoughts. What about all the others that go unnoticed all the time? Your brain is an invaluable tool that you can use to your advantage, so keep it filled with positive, proactive thoughts that will get you to where you want to go instead of in the other direction.

It is imperative that you continue to read, learn, and focus on health. Your mind moves in the direction of its most dominant thoughts, so fill it with good ones. The more you learn about health and fitness, the faster you will move toward a fit and healthy body. Think success, and you will be a success!

Know in your heart, soul, body, and mind that you are getting healthier every day, that you are already healthy, or that you are in the process of uncovering your own personal path to a healthier life. Constantly remind yourself how you will feel once you reach your goals. Visualize how your clothes will fit and imagine all the energy you will have once you get to your pinpointed destination.

Take at least fifteen minutes a day doing just that: visualizing your outcome to train your brain. Your brain does not know the difference between what you see with your eyes and what you imagine in your head. Remember the little guy upstairs taking notes all day? Well, every time you imagine yourself being healthy, that person is taking notes, and your body begins the process of moving toward that direction immediately.

Negative thoughts are just as powerful as positive ones, so keep thinking happy thoughts to stay in a positive frame of mind. Try this little experiment: remember a bad day you have had somewhere in the past. Now pay close attention to the way you felt emotionally and energetically; notice changes in your posture and body language. You may feel a sense of heaviness in your body, weighed down, sluggish, sad, or even angry. Now think about the best day of your life. Notice how it makes you feel positive, happy, physically lighter, and full of energy? Your body language changes, you stand taller, and even your facial expression is altered.

Mental imagery is a crucial part of the success puzzle; every successful person knows this and practices it, either consciously or subconsciously. That is why they are successful in the first place. I use this technique often, especially when preparing for something like a fitness competition. Surprisingly, when I spoke to competitors that consistently placed well, they confessed to using this technique too.

You are who you think you are, and who you think you are will have a bearing on your physiological and physical health. Your brain is so powerful that your thoughts can actually produce sickness and disease or health and vitality. Have you ever heard of women who believed that they were pregnant and actually developed body changes that made them appear as though they were pregnant even though they were not? What about monks in Tibet who control their body temperature and other bodily functions just by using thought? Did you know that people with multiple personalities may experience health problems during one personality but not another?

An article written in *The New York Times* health section on September 7, 2008, spoke of this phenomenon. The article talks about a gentleman by the name of Timmy who can drink orange juice while existing as Timmy, but as other personalities, if he drinks orange juice he gets hives, even though it is the same body. What is even more amazing about this particular story is that if Timmy drinks the juice and experiences no hives but changes personalities while the juice is being digested, he will get the hives. Then if the alternate personality is itching and broken out and the Timmy personality returns, the hives immediately disappear, along with the itching.

Doctors have noted many drastic biological changes with those patients that have multiple personalities when they switch from one personality to the next, including abrupt appearance changes; appearing and disappearing of rashes, welts, scars, wounds; handwriting and handedness changes; epilepsy; allergies; blood pressure; language; artistic talent; color blindness; and even change in the shape and curvature of the eye.

Medications will work differently from one personality to the next as well. Many times when a person experiences more than one personality, one or more of those personalities will be that of a child, and when that person is given a medication and the child personality arises, the medication will affect that person the same way it would affect a small child, even if it is given to an adult and responses are normal in the adult personalities. Researchers studying this phenomenon are working with multiple personality patients in an effort to learn more about the mind/body connection and the power that our thoughts have on our physical health.

Dr. Bennett Braun, a psychiatrist at Rush Presbyterian St. Luke's Medical Center in Chicago, said, "We're finding the most graphic demonstrations to date of the power of the mind to affect the body," and, "If the mind can do this in tearing down body tissue, I think it suggests the same potential for healing." Doctors are finding that the varying states of the mind actually change the body's biology and that people have a biological and psychological self, which work interdependently. As one changes, so does the other.

Remember that little person in your head, the one taking notes? Well, they also take notes on what they hear. So speak positively about yourself to others. Think and talk about yourself with respect and enthusiasm. Plus, make your internal dialog a cheerleader instead of a degrading jerk. What you think of yourself and say about yourself is what will eventually be.

How you view yourself is how others will view you as well. Fortunately or unfortunately, you are influenced by how your peer group views you, just as much as how you view yourself. If you convince them you are put together and on top of things, they will view you that way, and on days you do not necessarily feel that way, their expectations and view of you will bring you back up to the high status they hold in their mind. If you talk nasty about yourself, then your peer group will view you the same way you speak about yourself, and this can cause you to be locked into the stereotype you created in the first place, good or bad. It is a self-fulfilling prophecy, so make your prophecy a good one.

Set high standards for yourself and talk positively about you. Do not gloat; that is not attractive, but self-confidence is. Let the words that fleetingly visit your lips be that of self-respect and love for the most important person in your world, which is you. If you do this, then others around you will follow suit and do it too.

Parents do this all the time with their children by holding a high expectation of them and what they feel they can achieve. If you expect low standards, then you will get even lower than what you expect. If you expect great things, then even if you fall a little short, you will still achieve great heights. So expect great things, as well as speak and think highly of yourself always. Let your self-fulfilling prophecy be one of greatness and success.

ASSOCIATE EXERCISE WITH FUN

Unfortunately, many people associate exercise and general activity with work and unpleasant feelings. In reality, it is just an association people have that was made over time but one that is usually without merit.

If you sit around all day, do you feel lazy and tired or full of energy? Lazy and tired, right? What about if you spend a few hours participating in some fun activity with friends? You usually experience feelings of excitement, vitality, and generally have a fun time, right? So why is it that many people think of exercise as negative? It is just an association they have created in their head along the way that they believe and drives their behaviors. Therefore, to change their behaviors with regard to becoming more active, they will need to change their views and associations first.

This concept is not only true for activity and exercise but for eating better as well. So many people say to me that eating healthy is boring, bland, or it just does not taste as good. People complain that there are few healthy choices available to them, which makes it hard to eat better.

Change your life by changing the way you think. Evaluate the associations you already have about diet and exercise that may be inhibiting your progress. Start by making new associations regarding healthy eating and exercise with positive thoughts and feelings.

NO EXCUSES!

If your health is important to you, then *no excuses!*

- "I'm too busy."
- "I don't have time."
- "I have kids."
- "I work long hours."
- "I don't have time to eat breakfast or pack a lunch."
- "My mother is sick."
- "Life is too stressful."
- "I don't have the money."
- "I'll start next week, month, year, or when things slow down."
- "I don't have exercise equipment or a gym membership."

Excuses, excuses, excuses. Does this sound familiar? Trust me, I am just like you, and I make time. I have been a single mom for over twenty years. I run my own business, which equates to anywhere from forty to sixty hours a week. There are times when I am traveling three to four days a week and never home. I have two boys that go to sporting events, skating parties, birthday celebrations, and take up lots of my time. As far as money goes, there have been entirely too many times to count that I have had to steal from Peter, Paul, and John just to pay Ruth.

I think you get what I am trying to say here—stop with the excuses and make it work! If I can make time, you can make time. The key word here is *make.* You have to schedule it and make it a priority in your heart, soul, body, and mind, because you are the most important person in your universe!

Let me ask you this: what is your number one asset? The definition of an asset is something that brings you future economic benefit, something that makes you money. So what is it: your car, your house, your boat, your business, your job? No! It is *you!* Without you, there is nothing else. If you are sick, lacking in energy, not feeling up to it, stricken with disease, or dead, you will not be making very much money now, will you?

For all of you out there using your kids as an excuse, forget about it. You should be even more adamant about taking care of yourself. Your kids learn from you; they become mirror images of you and the way you live your life. Do you want your kids to be sick, overweight, tired, or stricken with disease when they are your age or younger?

Did you know that statistics forecast that one in every four people will develop type 2 diabetes in the next ten years, before the age of twenty? Do you want to be the one responsible for you or your child becoming diabetic or worse? Of course not.

Tough love is the answer; be tough about taking care of yourself and your family. Eat right, exercise, and use tough love. What I mean by tough love is stop making excuses and do what is good for you and your loved ones instead of what is easy. Stop taking the easy road and start taking the road less traveled; it is more scenic, fun, and rewarding, inside and out!

I have talked with a number of athletes throughout the years, and can you guess the average number of workouts they miss in a year? The answer I commonly get is none. Like Nike says, "Just Do It." Your goal should be to work out five days a week for at least an hour, regardless of what your goals are. It does not have to be some killer workout; just get off the couch and move your body.

I know what you're thinking: *But what if I'm on vacation?* or *What if I don't have exercise equipment?* The key is to move your body, and you can do that anywhere without any equipment. Use your body weight, walk up stairs, do jumping jacks and/or pushups, or march in place. Move any opportunity you get. If you're at work, instead of sending an e-mail, try walking over to your coworker, or taking the stairs instead of the elevator. Just stay as active as you can, and you will be implementing the same strategies that those successful at managing their weight do. Remember to keep your mind focused on little ways you can get more activity in each day. Even just simple movements can cause you to burn a few hundred calories, which can lead to pounds of fat over time.

PLANTING THE SEED

Another important aspect of getting fit is to surround yourself with fit people. If you hang around negative people that do not take care of their bodies, then neither will you. Remember the section regarding hanging out with a friend and subconsciously picking up on their words or actions? Well, there you go.

Surround yourself with people that will only help you to succeed and to become a better person. If you can pick up bad habits, then you can also pick up good ones. You can start surrounding yourself with fit people by sharing the wealth of your knowledge today. Tell everyone you know about this program and share it with him or her so you can make improvements together. By doing so, you will surround yourself with fit people, which will help to keep you motivated and on your path toward good health. Help to make the world a healthier place, because living in a healthier world will make your life easier too.

What could be more rewarding than spreading the seed of health? Watching loved ones make positive changes because you have is extremely rewarding, and I share that wisdom from personal experience. They may have noticed changes in your energy, attitude, weight, body composition, and more. Some may begin to change their lifestyle for competitive reasons, and that is okay, because you are planting the seed of health.

You will reap just as many rewards as them because you were the one to plant the seed that not only helped you grow but helped them grow as well. They will be thanking you for it later. In addition, it continues to keep you on track because they will be motivating you in return, at times when you may feel weak. You get back from life what you give; in other words, you reap what you sow.

ACTION GOAL: *FRAME OF MIND EXPERIMENT*

Think lean, mean, athletic machine.

That is exactly what you are, so believe it! Why do you think the army chants when they take their cadets on a run? Programming is the reason. They are programming their cadets when they are at their weakest point of mental resistance, which is during physical exhaustion.

Here is a little programming experiment to try. When you are exercising or relaxed, you are mentally more receptive to programming. So why not use this time to program yourself too? The next time you go for a walk or run, try doing just that. Chant something in your head or aloud that gets you motivated and pumped up to do more, go farther, and work harder. Think about how lean and mean you are or how invigorated you feel right at that moment.

Any motivating statements will do. Say it to yourself over and over again. Most of the time when a person works out, he/she thinks about how hard it is and how he/she really does not want to be exercising at all. Notice the difference in how you feel when you are chanting positively versus using negative internal or external dialog.

Try chanting something like, "I'm a lean, mean, athletic machine." A lot of top athletes do this. Look at Mohammad Ali; he spawned a popular phrase: "Float like a butterfly, sting like a bee." If you find a phrase that sparks some positive motivating feeling for you, then exercise becomes noticeably easier and a lot more rewarding inside and out.

STEP 2:

Goal Setting

How can you get somewhere if you don't know where you are going? What if you were the captain of a ship and it was your job to navigate the ocean in order to get your crew and passengers to a remote tropical island of paradise somewhere in the Pacific? The only problem is that you haven't been given the coordinates of where that island is, and the slightest turn in the wrong direction could take you hundreds of miles off course. You want to reach this island because you've heard it's paradise on earth. So you try asking around to see if anyone else has directions, but the directions you get are vague or are wrong because you are starting from a different point than what the directions explain. Regardless of the reason, if you do not have an actual address or point of destination for this island, well, you probably will never get there. What's worse is that you will probably be wandering around at sea feeling frustrated, angry, and hopeless.

To arrive at a destination, you need three distinct pieces of information:

- Where you're starting from
- Where you're going
- How to get there … exactly

Many people might know one or two of these pieces of information, but you have to know all three to reach a goal. For instance, you might know your home address, but if you don't know my grandma's, well, how will you get there? You need to know the precise ending point you aspire to achieve before you start out on your path to find it.

- Does this scenario sound familiar to you?
- Do you feel like you have been traveling in circles with your weight loss efforts and fitness efforts?
- Do you feel like you are getting vague instructions that are not completely suitable to what your situation or needs are, resulting in wasted time and energy due to heading in the wrong direction?
- Do you feel like there is some missing component or information that is preventing you from achieving permanent success?
- Are you confused about which way to turn or what active choice is best for you?

You need to know this: it's not your fault.

Seriously, there are so many ways to get to your ultimate weight- or fat-loss destination that not even the so-called "experts" can agree on the directions to get you there. Think about it: carb-free, fat-free, pineapples only, peanut butter diet, protein only, et cetera. If everyone has the same goal—weight or fat loss—why are there so many darn directions to get to there? Why are there so many weight loss products, exercise contraptions, and theories for attaining your perfect weight? And most importantly, what's right for you? Well, to answer that question, you have to answer a few questions first. Where are you now? Where do you want to go? How did you get where you are today? What path do you need to take or lifestyle changes will help you reach your fitness goals?

KNOW YOUR DESTINATION BEFORE YOU START YOUR JOURNEY

Maybe you have tried programs that ensure great results, and maybe you even achieved some initial results at first, but at some point in time, either those results were followed by rebound weight gain or failure to arrive at your ultimate desired outcome. Part of the problem lies in your lack of specificity of what it is that you really want and need.

Try this little experiment:

- Stand up.
- Lift one arm up and point to an object directly in front of you.

- Keep your feet planted firmly on the ground about a foot apart.
- Now rotate.

Were you successful in making it to your desired destination? You do not know because you were never given a pinpointed target to reach. It is impossible to know how far to turn or even where to turn if you do not have a predetermined goal in mind. Is this true with your weight loss and fitness goals as well?

Do you say things like, "I need to lose weight and get in shape," or "I need to start working out?" So if you drink a cup of coffee and drop one pound in water weight, you have accomplished your goal to lose weight, right? Not exactly! What exactly does "get in shape" *really* mean? Does it mean walking up a flight of stairs without being winded, or does it mean running five miles nonstop for you to consider yourself in shape? If you go to the gym one more day this year than last year, you have worked more, so I guess you accomplished that goal too, but is that going to get you the results you desire? Probably not.

Now try this:
- Stand up.
- Lift one arm up and point to an object directly in front of you.
- Keep your feet planted firmly on the ground about a foot apart.
- Rotate toward the right until you are pointing your finger 180 degrees in the opposite

direction to where you started, without moving your feet.

Were you successful this time in reaching your destination or goal? Yes, because you knew exactly what that goal was, where you were heading, and exactly what to do to reach it. You also had a specific and identifiable outcome in mind before you started the process, an outcome that you could visualize and then measure. If you were asked to go beyond your previously set goal, would you be able to do that as well? Yes, because once again you had a prior set specific goal in which to advance further. The key to constant improvement is setting goals, reaching those set goals, and then setting new ones that are beyond your prior achievements. This is how success is reached.

Before you leave this section, remember this: you have to know what you're aiming at in order to reach the target. Be specific about your weight loss and fitness-gain goals. Avoid general comments like:

- "Ugh, I need to get in shape."
- "I wish I was thinner."
- "I need to look better by summer."

Be more specific instead:

- "I would like to be able to run a mile without stopping by the end of the month."
- "I would like to lose ten pounds by the end of the summer."

- "I need to tone my abs over the next two months so I can see the line down the middle of my stomach or a six pack or two inches less in diameter."

Specificity is just one more way to think differently about your goals. In the past, you may have been too general to reach your goals. Again, it's not your fault. We are a culture plagued by indecision, generalities, and condescension. We say, "Get in shape," without really knowing what it means, but when you *Think Fit 2 Be Fit,* you *know* what "get in shape" means because you've specifically defined it.

Now you are free to reach your goals, once and for all!

WHAT ARE GOALS?

Setting personal goals is a critical step for succeeding in anything worth doing, be it professional, personal, and especially physical. So what are goals? Goals can be a number of things to a number of people. They can be statements of faith, a set of objectives, future conditions, expectations, ideals, a purpose to do something, a mission, or even a pinpointed destination.

Goals are obviously important, but why? Goals are important because they give you something to shoot for, a target, an end point, or a finish line; that "finish line" can be as simple as Grandma's house or losing five pounds, or as complicated as crossing the country or running a marathon.

Either way, goals help you maintain focus on difficult days, along with continued motivation as you accomplish each one. Goals also help you to identify dissatisfaction with your current fitness status. If you are unhappy with your current level of health and fitness, then you need to raise your bar of standards. A standard is a set of rules you consciously or unconsciously live by. One standard I set for myself is based on my physical appearance. One of my standards includes maintaining a specific amount of definition in my stomach area.

It is important for me, personally speaking, to be able to identify a defining line of separation down the center of my tummy and the outline of my two top quadrants of my abdominal muscles, which usually means for me that I have around 15 percent body fat. Consuming a poor diet reduces definition, causing my tone to decrease quickly. When this occurs, I know I have fallen below my bar of personal standards. This change in my physical appearance is a specific sign for me to clean up my diet by eating more natural, alive foods and exercising more.

Now don't get me wrong: I am *not* telling you this to make you feel bad about your physique if you do not have the same definition in your abs. My objective is to encourage you to think and be more aware of the standards you set for yourself. Are they specific enough for attaining your personal goals and the desired results you want? If you are not currently where you want to be when it comes to weight loss or fitness gain, then the answer is no.

Sometimes people set standards, but when they fall below those standards, they adjust them to compensate for the change instead of adjusting their life. A great example of this is when clothes start getting tight due to poor dietary choices and low activity levels, which is something that tends to happen to most people around the holiday season. When this happens, most people go buy bigger sizes instead of eating better and exercising more. They lower their standards over and over until eventually they are so completely unhappy with themselves that they feel it may be impossible to get back to where they once were. Setting goals raises your bar of standards and allows you to apply a proactive set of behaviors that help you to reach and maintain those goals successfully.

GOALS + ACTION = RESULTS

Have you set goals? This is a question that usually gets a very high "yes" response rate when I speak to classes all around the area. Have you set *specific* fitness and/or nutrition *goals?* Unfortunately, this question does not get as typically high of a response rate!

So if you know the importance of setting goals and you set goals in other aspects of your life, why is it that you do not set ones related to your health? Well, usually it's because you already know it but you are not feeling it. What I mean by that is that you *know* it in your head, you *know* what you need to do, but you do not have the proper motivation, knowledge, and/or understanding to do it. Most importantly, the feeling or emotional spark is missing, and it's that feeling or spark that makes you do something or not.

People say they know what they need to do all the time:

- I know I need to set goals ...
- I know I need to eat right ...
- I know I need to exercise ...
- I know I need to eat more veggies ...
- I know I need to drink more water ...
- I know I need to do ...
- I know I better try ...
- I know what I want ...

The problem is that most people do not follow through with action because it is only stuck in their heads, and for results to happen, you need to take that knowing and follow through with action. Action will get you purpose-driven results, and then you will not only know what to do mentally but you will feel it emotionally, spiritually, and physically.

Practicing something with action allows your whole being to feel the positive effects of that action, which perpetuates making proactive choices regularly easier and easier. You cannot just know something in your head; you need to feel it in your entire being, and once you do, especially if it is positive, you will want to continue doing it. This is why a proactive lifestyle is what gets you results.

Now that you know what goals are and why they are important, let's take a look at the process to setting and reaching them:

(1)   Identify the big picture.
(2)   Set detailed goals.
(3)   Map out your path.
(4)   Eliminate bricks.
(5)   Start now!
(6)   Reward yourself.

Step One: *Identify the Big Picture*

What is your "big picture" goal? Describe in detail your ultimate health and fitness goal. Be sure to use at least five to ten specific supporting details about this goal. For example, if your goal is to lose weight, try being more specific by giving exact numbers.

For instance, you may want to say, "My goal is to lose forty-two pounds. I want to reduce my waist size by fifteen inches. I want to have a waist circumference of thirty-eight inches. I want to wear size nine to ten pants and a medium-size shirt. I want to be at a healthy body fat for someone my age." Again, be very specific with your big picture goal or goals by using as many details as possible.

Use the space provided to write down some details about your own big picture goal:

_____

_____

_____

_____

_____

_____

_____

_____

_____

Now determine a reasonable date to reach this big picture goal or goals:

Date I want to reach my big picture goal:

_____

Step Two: *Setting Detailed Goals*

In this step, you will set up both long-term and short-term goals. Take a few moments to think about what your "big picture" goal is. Big picture goals are your ultimate or the sky-is-the-limit type of goals. These are long-term goals, which may take one to ten years to accomplish. Your big picture goal might be to obtain the perfect body you have always wanted, a specific clothing size or waist circumference, or your desired health and fitness level. It might be a specific accomplishment, like running a marathon or even climbing Mt. Everest. This is a special goal that you may have dreamed of for some time.

For me, this goal was to compete in fitness competitions and to be recognized for my accomplishments in a national fitness magazine. I first set this goal when I was about sixteen years old. I did not reach it until 2001 at the age of twenty-eight, more than twelve years later. I competed in the Women's Tri-Fitness (WTF) World, my very first competition, and placed first out of 144 girls in the skills division and eleventh overall. I was also recognized for some of my fitness and professional accomplishments in the *Oxygen* 2003 women's fitness magazine. The moral of the story is that you need to set your sails high and keep your eye on what it is that you really want. If you do, you will accomplish things you have never imagined you could.

Short-term goals are just that, smaller goals that are attained over a shorter period, which aid you in reaching your big picture goals. Short-term goals can be set for any length of time: daily, weekly, monthly, three-month, or even six-month intervals. Ideally, they should be attainable in a relatively short period, like a month, so that you are continually motivated toward reaching that ultimate goal.

The important thing to remember is that you can't have one without the other; short-term and long-term goals work together. First I set my big picture goal, but it was my short-term goals that kept me motivated. Sometimes it would take me months to perfect just one short-term goal, but the end results were worth it. These mini-goals not only kept me motivated, but they eventually led to my complete lifestyle and physical transformation. I was able to permanently change bad habits into new proactive ones that have lasted the entirety of my life.

Be specific when setting goals. If I told you that one of my goals was to have more energy and stamina, how would you be able to measure that? Be more specific. Rather than saying, "I need more energy and stamina," it is better to state something like, "I want to be able to walk three miles in sixty minutes and to maintain an exercise heart rate of 140 beats per minute for the duration of my workout." Of course, you need to have more energy and stamina to accomplish this if you are not already able to do so! The difference is now you have some *very specific criteria* for measuring progress. You need to start slow and move your way up, always developing and reaching for new goals.

The first and foremost step in developing your goals is to assess your current fitness level and identify the truth. Once you have finished this step, you will set up monthly goals for continued progress. In this section, list your areas of focus every month after you have assessed yourself.

Keep these goals posted in a viewable area, like on the fridge, next to the alarm clock, or on the bathroom mirror so you can be reminded of them each and every day. Whatever your mind is focused on, it will move toward attaining. This will produce continued motivation in making proactive choices that produce the results you desire. If your mind moves in the direction of its most dominant thought and you are thinking about health and fitness continually, then success is yours. The sky is the limit!

Step Three: *Map Out Your Path*

Remember our failed trip to that tropical island from the beginning of this chapter? How different would your journey have been if someone had simply drawn you a map to or given you navigational step-by-step directions?

Mapping out your path means setting up smaller short-term goals or checkpoints of measure for identifying change and creating change down your personal path toward health. If the little incremental changes you make produce no change at all, you can very easily adjust those mini-goals so that you start producing results as quickly as possible without losing too much time or motivation in the process. The goal is not to have you running a marathon by day two of your journey; the objective is to keep you moving forward *one tiny step at a time.*

When individuals take on too much by trying to reach too large an objective, it becomes overwhelming because to be successful you would have to change too much at one time in your current lifestyle and daily habits to accomplish such a feat. Breaking your larger goals up into tiny, easily reachable ones allows you to experience reoccurring joys of accomplishment on a regular basis. Feeling good about your mini-progresses will keep your motivational fire ignited so that you remain focused on plugging away toward the accomplishment of your big picture goals.

Using your big picture goal, develop three short-term goals that will aid you in accomplishing it. One short-term goal may be to lose a lesser amount of weight, like ten pounds in thirty days. Remember to be very specific and realistic:

Short-term goal #1:

_____

Short-term goal #2:

_____

Short-term goal #3:

_____

Next, choose three immediate changes that will help you reach these short-term goals. In other words, write down the actions you will take to reach these short-term goals. You may want to write down how often you are going to work out or make some specific, immediate changes to your diet. Once again, be very descriptive here.

A goal to "work out more" is simply not descriptive enough to reach your goals effectively. It doesn't give you an actual action to take. On the other hand, "working out five more minutes than I currently do" is more descriptive and will give you something specific to do. Try writing down the number of days, the duration of your workout, whether you are going to weight train or do aerobics, and what heart rate you will maintain during the duration of your workout.

Immediate change #1:

_____

Immediate change #2:

_____

Immediate change #3:

_____

Step Four: *Eliminating Bricks from Your Wall of Despair*

Let's take some time now to get rid of all those excuses you have by bringing them to light. One excuse I often hear is the time excuse: "I don't have time to work out." Now, I know this is not as true as you might think. Why?

Well, do you watch TV or read the newspaper? First, watching TV or reading the newspaper is never going to create a healthy body by any means, nor is it going to help you reach your personal health and fitness goals.

Secondly, if you exercise during commercials, you can get in as much as twenty minutes of exercise for every hour of TV watched. You can also read while riding a stationary bike or walking on the treadmill, which is a proactive way to accomplish your goals while doing other things you enjoy.

To get specific about your excuses and how you can overcome them, list at least ten different excuses you use regularly, such as "not having enough time" or "not having a gym membership." Next, turn it into a proactive statement that changes your perspective and helps you reach your purpose instead.

For instance, if you watch TV each night yet you say you do not have time, explain how you can change that into a positive. Turn this around by stating that you will walk up and down the stairs nonstop during commercials instead of just sitting on the couch:

Excuse	Why is it an excuse?
Example: _I don't have enough time_	_I can create time by exercising in between commercials_
(1) _____	_____
(2) _____	_____
(3) _____	_____
(4) _____	_____
(5) _____	_____
(6) _____	_____
(7) _____	_____
(8) _____	_____
(9) _____	_____
(10) _____	_____

Step Five: *Start Now*

Start taking action immediately!

In the goal section, you wrote down some immediate changes you will start right away. Choose one of those immediate modifications, put this book down right now, and *go do it.* You can come back and finish once you have completed this task.

Waiting only delays success. Do not fall into the trap of doing it when you feel like doing it because feelings always follow actions. Remember the old saying, "An object in motion stays in motion?" Well, if your body starts moving, it wants to keep moving, and what follows are "feel-good" feelings.

Think about it: when you sit down, your body wants to stay down. Most people that work all day sitting at a computer want to come home and sit some more because their body has been doing it already and wants to continue doing it. It takes a lot more energy to get an object moving than it does to keep it moving, so get up and do something to begin reaching your goals now!

Step Six: *Reward Yourself*

You reward your family, kids, friends, and coworkers regularly, but do you reward yourself? Do you ever just pat yourself on the back or do something special for yourself? Unfortunately, probably not as often as you should, and when you do reward yourself, it is usually negative reinforcement.

I see it time and time again, where people reward themselves for exercising, eating well, and losing weight with a huge bowl of ice cream. Doesn't quite make sense now, does it? You are working hard, making positive, proactive changes, and then your efforts are sabotaged by eating ice cream or some other junk food of choice. Now you are right back where you started.

Choose positive reinforcements instead. Try treating yourself to a trip to the mall for some new clothes, to a day at the spa, with some new cool tool or sporting good you've been wanting. Positive reinforcement is a fun way to stay motivated toward reaching your goals over time. Reward does not always have to be something tangible either.

What is your internal dialog? Is it positive or negative? Do you beat yourself up or pat yourself on the back while saying to yourself, *"Way to go! Nice job, you did it!"* Just like in the real world, we like it when someone pays us a compliment, so take the time to notice all of your little accomplishments along the way, and instead of beating yourself up for not being perfect, say something good inside that head of yours.

List thirty rewards that you can choose from for each time you reach one of your goals. Be sure to have a wide variety of gifts to choose from, and try matching the size of your reward with the size of your accomplishment. I mean, you would not take a trip to Hawaii each and every time you ate all your vegetables, but you might take a trip to Hawaii if you lost one hundred pounds.

Choose small rewards for small accomplishments and big rewards for big accomplishments. Be creative with your reward list. One idea may include giving yourself an hour of time to do whatever you want like: visit a friend, take a candlelit bubble bath, go for a walk in the park, see that movie you've been wanting to, take a day trip with the guys, et cetera. For your big picture goal, choose an incredibly exciting reward so reaching that goal is worth it in many ways. Be sure to choose positive, proactive choices that support your efforts as a whole.

(1) _____

(2) _____

(3) _____

(4) _____

(5) _____

(6) _____

(7) _____

(8) _____

(9) _____

(10) _____

(11) _____

(12) _____

(13) _____

(14) _____

(15) _____

(16) _____

(17) _____

(18) _____

(19) _____

(20) _____

(21) _____

(22) _____

(23) _____

(24) _____

(25) _____

(26) _____

(27) _____

(28) _____

(29) _____

(30) _____

PARTING WORDS ABOUT GOAL SETTING

Now that you know where you are and where you are heading, it is time to look into how you got here in the first place. To do this, you had to first to understand how the most powerful machine in the world works—that machine is your brain. Understanding what you think, why you think a particular way, how your thinking creates who you are, and how to use the power of thought to change your life is what you will continue to learn throughout this book.

Before moving forward, take a closer look at what you have learned this week and put it into practice for a full week's time before moving on. This will ensure retention and more successful action toward embedding this material into your lifestyle permanently. Implement the goals you have set in this step and practice your new healthy habits daily to ensure results.

STEP 3:

Understanding Nutrition

When we take a look at the definition of the word *nutrition*, we find that it means the ingredients or necessary nutrients it takes to create, build, and keep your body healthy. In other words, you truly are what you eat. When it comes to nutrition, try thinking of it in terms of bodybuilding, not in the normal sense of the word, but in the way of building the body's health.

BE A BODYBUILDER—LITERALLY!

I have always kind of thought of myself as a bodybuilder, even though I'm not one of those people that get really huge and muscle-bound like you see on the covers of fitness magazines. But I am a bodybuilder in the sense that my main focus from nutrition is to *build the body* I want, in the same way you build anything in life.

If you want to bake a cake, there are specific ingredients that you need in order to make it. You can't make cake out of dirt and worms and expect it to be cake, just like you can't eat unhealthy foods and expect to build a healthy body. Food is only meant as fuel for your body for the ability to perform all of the daily functions necessary and the most important building block for creating the body you want and desire.

Too many people use food as a form of entertainment instead of seeing it as a necessity for health and vitality. If you view food as an added form of entertainment, then you are more likely to make poor decisions when it comes to the selections that you put into your mouth. Food should be enjoyable, absolutely, but in a healthful way.

The wrong foods can be very addictive and create negative results in your body. Eating unhealthy choices regularly causes you pain and agony at some point after its consumption, either in higher blood sugar, excess weight, a "high" or a "low," et cetera. Instead of choosing food as entertainment for your tongue, try hanging out with friends and family, or do something exciting for the heart, soul, body, and/or mind as a source of entertainment instead.

You can even use food to bring people together and have fun, but choose healthy alternatives instead of the old, unhealthy, highly processed, sugary snacks of the past. Consume food with the concept that it is nourishment for the body, and choose to consume things that will make you feel good because you are building better health and a better body.

This bodybuilding concept helped me on many a tough occasion when temptation was luring me into eating unhealthy stuff that I'd only regret later. During those tough times, I'd simply remind myself that food is meant for building the body I want, and with that in mind, I needed to make the best choice for doing that if I wanted to reach my goals. Over time, this concept became embedded in my normal thinking habits about food, and instead of being tempted every day to make bad choices, I was almost always able to make good decisions. And if a day comes along where I slip and stray away from my good eating habits—for instance, when there is a special event like a wedding—I recognize it for what it is and get back on track immediately. I don't beat myself up about it; instead, I start where I left off and continue to recognize all of the positive choices I've been making.

FAD DIETS ARE EVENTS, NOT LIFESTYLES

When it comes to eating healthy, there is a lot of conflicting information out there today, especially myths that are usually created by fad diets. We are bombarded every season with new fad diets, from the South Beach Diet to the Lemonade Diet. The list is endless.

Millions of people just like you try the hottest diet on the market, hoping this will be the one that finally works, but it ends up working like the rest of the diets you have tried in the past, and eventually, you find yourself searching for another. These diets usually provide some results, like quick weight loss, but unfortunately, it is never a permanent solution.

The weight loss attained on these diets isn't usually maintained; otherwise, you might not be reading this book. More often than not you gain it all back, along with a few extra pounds to go with it. I know because before I started eating the way I describe in this book, I did too.

Remember, health and fitness is a lifestyle, not an event. Fad diets are events; they are here for a short duration but are never a permanent solution to your ongoing weight-management problems. Unless you want to live on a restricted diet for the rest of your life, that is. I know I can't, nor do I want to. I like food, all different kinds of it, so even the thought of restricting myself in any way seems barbaric. Just remember, if a fad diet really worked, then America would not be getting fatter each year.

Well, if you're with me, then that means you will need to learn how to eat in a way that is satisfying, enjoyable, good for your health, and that gets you the results you want and deserve; in other words, a lifestyle. Eating with these four goals in mind is the only way you will ever stick to a healthy nutritional plan.

The concepts outlined in this book are the steps I have used personally to reach my fitness goals and the fundamentals that were necessary for me to be able to get onto the fitness competitor stage, as well as featured in *Oxygen* magazine. I have also taught these same principles to my clients over the years, which equated to great success for them as well. There are many tips that you'll be able to use for tweaking your own nutritional and exercise regimens, which will help you finally attain your personal goals for good.

Use the nutritional tips in the upcoming pages to create a proactive lifestyle that will lead you to positive change in your overall health that lasts. Just remember, when you are doing it the right way, it is easily attained and the results keep coming, but it happens over time. Eating well produces physical and physiological changes that are gentle and natural for the body.

When something is good for you, it feels good when you are doing it. On fad diets, you normally feel like you're missing out on something; your diet is restricted in some way and not balanced. It's not fun. Therefore, in the end, you quickly return to your prior eating habits happily because of all the negative feelings that you were experiencing by eating in an unbalanced way.

You won't feel that way here, not with my program. My program entails step-by-step changes that you will easily make over time, which will help you reach your goals in a deliberate, aware manner and with excitement. You will see, just as I did, how your body and overall health change with each step toward the body of your dreams. The best part about how my program will help you is that it's not a quick fix, so the results last a lifetime.

THE SEVEN BASIC COMPONENTS OF NUTRITION

What I learned over the years is that diet is one-third of the fat-loss equation. With all the hype on fad diets, it can be confusing as to what and how much you should be eating. There are seven basic components that comprise a well-developed nutritional program:

(1) Protein
(2) Carbohydrates
(3) Dietary Fiber
(4) Vitamins
(5) Minerals
(6) Fats
(7) Water

A well-balanced diet has one primary purpose: to provide life for your body. The purpose for the food you eat is for building, repairing, and providing you with energy for bodily and everyday functioning. Knowing this helped me to continue looking at food in a bodybuilding way, and I believe it will help you too. Eating healthy and creating the body you want is about mastering the fundamentals, not about the new and greatest pill or diet on the market.

It's the simple yet profound fundamentals of nutrition that give you the body you desire and build health. When your diet isn't comprised of the right balance of these seven elements, then your physiology becomes imbalanced, and the result is undesirable weight. Knowing and understanding how these seven components help you to "build your body healthy" is the foundation of being and living fit. This knowledge will give you the power to choose foods that provide maximum benefits and create maximum results naturally, literally the way nature intended.

This chapter will help you gain a basic understanding of what the seven fundamental nutrients are, their general physiological effects in the body, why they are important in the health-building process, and how they aid in helping you attain your weight loss and personal fitness goals. This is where I started my path to better eating and where your path begins as well.

The First Fundamental: *Protein*

THE HEALING POWER OF PROTEIN

As I gradually learned more about eating in a proactive way, I realized from all the reading and questioning I was personally doing that protein had to be a major component in my daily diet. Coming from a family where bread, pasta, and other white flour products were the most prevalent foods in our diet made this step one of the more difficult changes for me to make. I mean, we were eating bread with our pasta or bread with mashed potatoes during the same meal. Actually, now that I realize it, most people reading this right now might ask, "What's wrong with that?"

Unfortunately, it's not a balanced meal. It's all energy food that is usually being eaten at a time of the day when you don't need much energy, like dinnertime. Adding more protein wasn't the hard part; it was eliminating white flour products, and especially bread, from my diet.

I was like, "What, no bread? Are you kidding me?" A major part of the problem was that I needed to rethink the way I ate at all of my meals, especially since all of them consisted of these types of foods—and lots of them!

I felt like if I eliminated white flour products, especially bread, from my diet altogether, I wouldn't have much left to eat. I continued to focus on purposeful eating, which changed my perspective. What I mean by purposeful—or purpose-driven—eating is that you eat with a *specific purpose* or outcome in mind. Instead of focusing on what I couldn't have, I began to focus on what *would* help me get the results I wanted.

Proteins and veggies were where I looked, and over time I eventually trained myself to think differently about my meal compositions. In the end, my meals became more exciting and tasteful than they had ever been; this only motivated me to continue making more positive changes elsewhere in my diet.

Incorporating this as a permanent adjustment in my diet took about six months to do. It was actually more difficult from a mental aspect than a physical one. Physically I felt great, and almost immediately my body started changing for the better. I looked more toned than I had ever been, and for the first time in my life, I thought I just might be able to compete at some point in the future.

Now I eat that way all the time, and for the most part, it's a habit. In other words, I do it without even thinking about it. It's so ingrained into my lifestyle (habitual) that it is part of who I am and how I eat all the time.

Let's take a look at why protein is so important when you are trying to build a healthy body. Protein is the body's major building material. The brain, muscles, and other bodily tissues, such as skin and hair, are all made primarily of protein.

Interestingly enough, if you're not getting enough protein now, you may notice that your nails and hair are weak and brittle. As I increased the protein in my diet, I noticed almost immediately that my hair and nails grew faster and looked healthier too. Protein is also used to make a multitude of different types of cells, including enzymes and hormones, which regulate bodily processes, such as digestion and water balance.

Most people are unaware that protein also plays an important role in fighting off sickness and disease because it is a necessary component for building anti-bodies, which are the cells in your body that fight off foreign organisms that would normally lead to sickness and disease.

Symptoms of an inadequate amount of protein in your diet may include frequent colds or flu, malnutrition, brittle hair and nails, hair loss, decreased hair pigmentation, Meuhrcke's lines (white marks/lines on nails), edema, skin hyperpigmentation, certain types of dermatitis, exacerbated acne problems, delayed healing or inability to heal wounds, bed sores, along with muscle weakness or wasting.

Interestingly, ever since I increased the protein in my diet, I don't get as sick as often, or, when I do get sick, I don't get hit as hard as I used to when growing up. Once, I even worked with a client that had terrible acne well into her adult years, and the problem with this was that a small pimple would turn into a large sore that just wouldn't heal. She was a vegetarian, and after reviewing her diet, I found that she was getting little to no protein in her daily diet. I recommended that she start taking a protein supplement to balance out her nutritional plan and enhance her training program. My suggestion was that she start with three to four servings of twenty grams of protein a day.

Unfortunately, she ignored my advice initially, and her symptoms continued. This particular client was also having some other medical problems that necessitated a visit to her primary care physician, who ordered blood tests and found that her amino acids (what actually make up protein in your body) were at critically low levels. The doctor told her that if they were any lower they would have to put her in the hospital because other life-threatening complications could arise.

This same doctor had also suggested that she consume three to four servings of protein a day via a whey protein supplement to balance out her diet, the same suggestion I had made. Within several weeks of taking my advice, she noticed her energy levels had increased dramatically, and the acne on her face had almost completely disappeared.

She stopped getting the sores on her face from ruptured zits that weren't healing, and her acne never got as bad as it had in the past again.

Remember, it's not all about weight; eating right benefits the whole body, and when your body is healthy, your life is healthy. (We're building the body healthy, remember?) Protein is a vital nutrient, and getting an adequate amount in your diet can also enhance other areas of your health involving mental, emotional, and physical well-being. Therefore, it is crucial to make sure you consume several servings a day for balanced nutrition.

To drive the point home even further, I'd like to share a story I heard at a lecture that completely changed my views on the importance of protein. I had the pleasure of attending a lecture presented by the father of protein supplements, Dr. Scott Connelly. Dr. Connelly is the creator of a bioengineered food product that became the world's top supplement line called MET-Rx.

It was his work with burn victims in the intensive care unit at Massachusetts General Hospital that got him started researching the role protein played in the healing process. During his presentation, he showed slides of a patient that was admitted with third-degree burns over 75 percent of his body. The relatively thin victim, the doctor explained, had been receiving ten thousand calories a day over a thirty-day period before he finally died of starvation. Having the patient die of starvation left the doctor and his colleagues at a loss as to the cause. How could someone literally starve to death when their body was receiving over ten thousand calories a day?

In his research, Dr. Connelly found that the body uses nitrogen in the healing process, which is a byproduct produced in the breakdown of protein. Nitrogen is utilized by the body for healing soft tissues, open wounds and cuts, colds, to develop antibodies for fighting viruses, and much more. Your body can break down the protein that you ingest from the foods you eat, or it can break down the protein from which your muscles are made. If you do not ingest enough protein in your diet, as with the burn victim, your body will break down your own muscle tissue and use what it needs to commence healing. The ten thousand calories a day the burn victim was receiving was from glucose water, which did not give him the adequate protein/nitrogen needed for healing, and therefore, his body literally ate away at his muscle tissue in an effort to get enough healing nutrients for repair.

The victim's body continued breaking down his muscle mass in an effort to supply the body with the necessary nutrients needed for recovery, but because his diet was deficient in protein, this process continued until, eventually, normal vital functions ceased to operate and death resulted.

If you do not get enough of this important nutrient in your diet, you will break down your own muscle as well, inhibiting successful weight loss and fitness success. MET-Rx got its start as a prescribed nutrient for healing, from Dr. Connelly to his patients that were experiencing difficulty in wound healing. When bodybuilders caught wind of these breakthroughs, they started using his products themselves, and MET-Rx was born; the rest is history.

Ideally, to remain in a positive nitrogen balance, to give your body what it needs, and to aid in your body-building efforts, you will need to eat several servings of protein frequently throughout the day. Peter W.R. Lemon, PhD, director of the exercise nutrition research laboratory at Canada's University of Western Ontario, found that individuals actually need as much as 1.6–1.8 g/kg, or 0.7–0.8 grams per pound of body weight. So if your goal is weight loss, why should you be so concerned about protein, other than for healing purposes? Well, let's take a look at that next.

MUSCLE DRIVES YOUR METABOLISM (AND PROTEIN DRIVES MUSCLE)

One of the number one concepts that I learned about early in my career and bodybuilding process is that *muscle drives your metabolism*. Therefore, the more muscle you have, the more calories you will burn all day, every day. This was a challenging concept for me to wrap my head around initially, especially as a woman that only wanted to get leaner. The concept of getting leaner or more toned for a woman usually means they want to be smaller.

The challenge for me was trying to understand how adding more muscle to my body would help me accomplish this idea of getting more toned *and* smaller. As you will see later in the book, muscle takes up less room than fat when compared in pounds. Therefore, adding muscle and burning more calories on a consistent basis helped me to burn off the fat that was already stored on my body while creating a more toned appearance. In the end, I actually weighed more but wore a smaller size in clothing.

Healthy muscle increases the efficiency of your fat burning capabilities because it takes much more energy to maintain and keep alive than fat does. In fact, it has been estimated that for each pound of muscle you have on your body, you will burn approximately thirty to fifty calories a day. Professional bodybuilders, due to their massive size related to extra lean muscle, may need to consume as many as ten thousand or more calories a day just to maintain their size.

If you add ten pounds of muscle to your body, then you will be burning anywhere from three hundred to five hundred additional calories a day. That is nine thousand to fifteen thousand calories a month, which equates to three to four pounds of fat loss in thirty days, or thirty-six to forty-eight pounds of fat loss a year. Wow, imagine how great that would be, instead of gaining the national average of 3.2 pounds of body weight and excess fat every year. I can tell you that I've worn a size five for more than fifteen years consistently. Yet we are programmed to believe that weight gain is an inevitable part of life, which it is if you eat poorly, but if you eat to build your body healthy, it isn't.

Did you know that between proteins, fats, and carbo-hydrates, protein is the most difficult nutrient to digest? You can actually increase your metabolism by 25 percent during digestion of this important nutrient. In other words, 25 percent of the calories you consume from protein are burned up in the process of breaking it down into a usable resource for your body. What an easy way to burn a few extra calories!

Fat and carbohydrates only use up about 10 percent of their total ingested calories during metabolism. Protein is not stored in the body, like fat and carbohydrates are, so it is important to eat protein rich sources frequently throughout the day. Based upon the previously mentioned research, a minimum of two to four servings, approximately twenty to thirty grams/serving, is the minimal suggested amount for optimal health. Try to include some protein with every meal and at least one of your snacks to reach this daily goal. If you're not getting much protein in your diet currently, then start by adding a serving to one of your meals while lessening or eliminating some of the carbs you may be consuming at that meal, especially later in the day.

It's all too common that people choose to eat two different starch selections at dinner, so this might be the best meal to start with when making this change. That way, you will not be increasing the calories you are consuming; instead, you'll only be exchanging one source of nutrients for another.

In the end, because protein is harder to break down, it will be like you are getting fewer calories, but you will feel more fulfilled after your meal because blood sugar levels will remain more level. The key is to make simple changes that are easy to live with when making adjustments to your meal menu.

Start with one meal and then work your way up to two or three meals until your entire meal plan is revamped. After each change, pay close attention to the way you feel and how your body looks for the next few weeks after making the change. For me, eliminating breads and adding two to four servings of protein to my diet each day worked wonders. My body really began to transform after this change, more than it had ever changed in the past. Balance is the key, so eating all protein and little to no carbohydrates is neither healthy nor balanced. The goal is to enhance your nutritional plan with each change, not create imbalance or scarcity.

PROTEIN SUPPLEMENTS

Protein sources include naturally lean meats, poultry, fish, nuts, seeds, legumes, and eggs, as well as soy foods. There are also a number of excellent protein supplements on the market to help fulfill your protein needs, if you find that getting enough of this nutrient is a challenge. When choosing a protein supplement, pick one low in carbohydrates, especially low in added sugars. There are several varieties on the market that use Stevia, a natural sweetener, which does not affect blood sugar or insulin levels and is a more ideal choice, in my opinion, for those interested in eating a clean and healthy diet. I do supplement with a whey protein powder that is 100 percent natural. Keep in mind that it is always best to get your nutrient sources from whole, natural foods first than from supplements, but with today's busy schedules, sometimes it is not always possible.

When choosing protein supplements, look below at the types of supplements, which are listed in the order of my highest preference first:

- Protein drinks and powders tend to be low in carbohydrates and have little added sugars or artificial sweeteners. I always encourage you to choose a natural variety over one that has added artificial ingredients, especially one with added artificial sweeteners, as an effort to keep your diet clean and as close to natural for the body as possible.

- Meal replacements, such as the Myoplex or MET-Rx packets, may or may not be low in added sugars. They are usually somewhere around equal in carbohydrates and tend to be high in protein (around twenty to forty grams) per serving. This type of protein supplement has a good balance of fats, proteins, and carbohydrates and is usually higher in calories as well. Because carbohydrates are more easily accessible than proteins from normal food choices, these types of supplements should be used in place of a meal, instead of added to or in between meals. These supplements are great for those individuals that tend to skip meals due to a busy lifestyle or that need something quick, which also keeps them on track with their fitness goals.

- Protein bars should be a last resort when it comes to getting lean, due to the quality of protein used and other additives that make them taste better. In fact, when competing, it's one of the first things that I and most other competitors eliminate from their diets; otherwise, it's impossible to get a lean as you need to for the event. Again, if you have a tendency to skip meals or are looking for something sweet to munch on, bars can be a better choice than other high sugary junk food. I would encourage you to view them more as a "cheat treat," for the most part.

LEAN PROTEIN SOURCES AND SERVING SIZES

20–30 grams = Serving Size

Meat, Fish, Eggs, Poultry
3–4 oz = serving size
Size of the palm of your hand in diameter
and 1 inch thick

Protein Drinks
1–1 1/2 scoops
20–30 grams

Grade A = Best Protein Sources
Poultry, Fish, Lean Beef, Egg Whites

Grade B = Mediocre Protein Sources
Protein supplements (must be high protein and very low carbs to be considered—protein drinks), soy products (unsweetened soy milk and tofu)

Grade C = Low Quality Protein Sources
Dairy products, nuts, other soy products, protein supplements (bars and drinks high in carbs)

The Second Fundamental:
Carbohydrates

Carbohydrates are usually the most prevalent food source in most everyone's diet, as it was once in mine. When changes are made to your diet regarding this nutrient, however, the results can be amazing. It was eliminating highly processed, poor carbohydrate choices and replacing them with better quality, high-fiber, whole grain carbs that helped me attain my goals faster and with a lot more ease.

Remember, we are not eliminating any of these seven nutrients; you need them all, so in no way am I suggesting you kick carbs altogether. Instead, the key is choosing better carb selections, as well as making sure you aren't getting in too many carbohydrates in general to produce great results.

For instance, I eliminated all white flour products and Americanized wheat flour products. What I mean by "Americanized" is that products will say they are whole grain or whole wheat, but when you read the labels, it says that the product used enriched wheat flour, which usually means that the whole wheat was bleached—removing twenty-six different nutrients or more in the process—therefore, it needed to be re-enriched. Unfortunately, when it's re-enriched, only about four to six nutrients are added back in.

You can usually tell which products are Americanized or not. For instance, when looking at bread products, if the bread is light and fluffy, it's not really the type of product that you want to add into your diet. Light and fluffy bread is too well-refined and acts like sugar in the bloodstream because it's so easily broken down that it causes spikes in your blood sugar levels. These spikes in blood sugar levels are one of the reasons why you get cravings and want to eat more and more carbs. One of the first things I noticed once removing bread products from my diet was that I didn't get the cravings for white flour or bread products like I did in the past. This only made eating well a lot easier to do.

In the world of fitness competitors, bread is an absolute no-no and one of the top things to eliminate if you are serious about competing. Even if you aren't competing but just want to lose weight or look like you compete or could be in a magazine, eliminate all white flour products from your diet for some amazing results.

If you're going to have any, then have them on a cheat day. Think of it like this: the only real difference between bread, donuts, cake, and cookies is the sugar content. Light, fluffy bread is just cake with less sugar. Now, if that's true, then why would you eat it several times a day if you're trying to attain a lean physique? You wouldn't, I don't, and most competitors don't either. It will be a challenge making this change in your diet, but it's well worth it in the end.

The immediate and most important function of carbohydrates is to supply continuous energy to the body. In other words, if protein is the building blocks for the body, then carbs are fuel for the body. Foods rich in carbohydrates can be found mainly in plant sources like wheat, which is used for making breads and pastas, as well as other food products.

Foods classified as carbohydrate rich foods include choices such as rice, pasta, yams, potatoes, beans, lentils, bagels, oatmeal, fruits, vegetables, sugar, fructose, dextrose, honey, et cetera.

Carbohydrates are a necessary component to your fat-loss program, but choosing the right carbs is the key. When you accomplish this feat, you can increase your energy levels, elevate your mood, prevent major emotional swings, and keep your hunger in check as well. Our modern day diet consists mostly of highly processed carbohydrates, so eliminate the processed ones and replace them with less processed, whole grain versions. Not the types of carbs that say "whole grain" on the box but are a lot like the highly processed ones. Choose whole grain versions where you can see the whole grains with your eyes and feel the difference in your mouth.

One of the number one things I learned about being fit is that the closer a food is to being picked fresh from the vine, the better it is for your body. Fresh foods have more naturally occurring nutrients in them, and they are what the body needs. Whole, natural foods should compose the majority of your dietary choices, so try reducing and eventually eliminating all processed carbs for best results; if I can do it, then you can too. I understand that this is a very challenging feat to accomplish, but I can tell you it was one of the best things I have ever done for myself.

The results were spectacular, both physically and energetically. Try it, and you will be amazed yourself, as I was, at how you feel. I can tell you that as each year passes I feel better, more alive, and healthier overall then I did at twenty years of age, and you can too. Just try it and you'll see.

CRAVINGS

Knowing how food affects you on a physiological level is an important step in understanding why you get cravings. Cravings are not just bothersome urges, like a little devil sitting on your shoulders telling you, "Do it, come on, go ahead and eat that chocolate cake," just to keep you from reaching your weight loss goals. Cravings are temptations driving you to take action due to a deficiency your body is feeling and desperately trying to get you to fill. Pregnant women, for example, have been known for their outrageous cravings, including cravings for dirt or nonfood items known as "pica." *Disgusting,* you might say, but this bizarre behavior is easily recognized by doctors as a mineral deficiency, and dirt is filled with minerals.

The most common cravings I encounter with clients are cravings for sweets. There are three major reasons why you may have a sweet tooth:

(1) The first is dehydration. Sweets, which are mostly comprised of sugar, are classified as simple carbohydrates. Carbohydrates "hydrate" the body. If you look up the word *carbohydrate*, you'll find that it means "watered carbon," or carbon with attached water molecules. For example, the formula for glucose (which is what table sugar is comprised of) is $C_6H_{12}O_6$. If you think back to high school science class, you'll remember H_2O was the molecular formula for water. Looking at the glucose formula, you see the similar hydrogen-oxygen mix that water has. When you are low in water or dehydrated, consuming carbohydrates is one way for your body to get the water it needs fast. Unfortunately, you also get a lot of unwanted and empty calories that come along with it, which leads to excess body fat and weight gain. This is also true for those who crave salt. Salt pulls water into the body, but when the excess salt leaves the body, it takes water with it. The result is that you end up more dehydrated than before you started.

(2) The second reason why you may crave sweets is your body is low in energy, or the fuel it needs to function. Due to today's hectic schedules and long hours, you may find it very difficult to eat frequently enough throughout the day to sus-

tain your body's energy needs, and eating a big meal at seven o'clock at night isn't helping you for that low energy feeling at noon, seven hours earlier. It's important to eat a little something healthy every three to four hours to keep your blood sugar and energy levels where they need to be to maintain your current level of activity throughout the day, and that means mental activity too. When your body drops below minimal energy needs, it will respond with the physiological effects that you feel as a craving. Why? Not eating causes low blood sugar levels, and when blood sugar levels are low, your body needs energy quickly to elevate these blood sugar levels back to normal. You do not expect your car to run on empty, so why would you expect your body to?

(3) The third reason why you may crave sweets is related to eating high glycemic foods in the first place. High G.I. foods throw off your blood sugar levels, causing peaks then valleys. When sugar levels become too low after a spike, cravings are triggered, which is a sign for you to eat something and bring them back to normal. Candy and highly processed foods are those types of carbs that will cause these types of changes in blood sugar levels and, therefore, produce cravings. Skipping meals can also lead to low blood sugar, which will cause cravings and can lead you to binge. Grazing or eating

small amounts of healthy treats throughout the day will prevent this from happening. As you can see, cravings are a vicious cycle, and the only way to stop the cycle is to drink lots of water (shoot for a gallon a day), eat better quality carbohydrates like fruits, vegetables, and whole grain, high-fiber versions, and stay away from high sugar treats in the first place.

WHAT'S PROCESSED?

Processed food encompasses everything that is not picked from a vine. If it does not resemble food grown in a garden or a freshly cut piece of meat, fish, or poultry, or if it has more than one ingredient, then it is considered processed.

The more a food is processed, the worse it is for your body. For the most part, it halts progress when it comes to weight loss. And if that does not deter you, then maybe the fact that they can be harmful or toxic to your body will, and a diet high in these types of foods may inevitably lead to disease. A great example of how poor choices in one's diet can cause debilitating health problems, even for someone young and in good physical condition, is presented in the documentary of Morgan Spurlock's *Super Size Me*.

This incredible documentary of a guy eating three meals a day from a fast-food restaurant supplies the viewer with some profound information regarding how the foods you eat affect your health and can even cause drug addictive-like effects in your body. In the documentary, professionals from Harvard University discuss the effects of how some foods can actually respond in ways that create an opiate effect in the brain and how opiate-blocking drugs, normally used in rehabilitation for drug addiction, can actually eliminate cravings and drug effects of those foods. One professional gives an example of how, when taking such opiate-blocking drugs, a chocolate addict will actually no longer crave chocolate, even if it is placed right in front of him or her.

It is the physiological effects in your system that actually cause you to crave specific foods after eating them, and these are the same foods that are abundant in just about every young person's diet today. Overeating is another problem created by processed foods, which, due to the low-fiber and nutritional contents of these foods, along with their addictive properties, cause the consumer to eat more, even when they are not hungry.

Some examples of processed carbs are:

- Breads:
  - White bread, French bread, bagels, highly processed wheat bread
  - Products made with enriched wheat flour
- Pasta:
  - Spaghetti, macaroni
  - Any type pasta made with white flour; even wheat pasta is not the most desirable form of whole grain that you can choose from
- Cereals:
  - Corn Flakes, Special K, Raisin Bran,

most children's cereals, and any cereals
that have added sugars or enriched flour
- Snack Foods:
  ° Potato chips, fat-free cakes, cookies,
  crackers, fat-free ice cream or yogurt that
  have added sugars or artificial sweeteners

A processed food is basically anything that comes in a box, bag, or is prepared.

BE A LABEL LEARNER

Have you ever read some of the labels of the foods you eat? Do you know what all those ingredients are? Some are too difficult to even pronounce, let alone digest. Always remember, when it comes to food and the number of ingredients it has, less is best. Use herbs to spice up dishes and natural sweeteners, like fruit, to sweeten your food.

Think picked from the vine, freshly grown, or one-ingredient foods. In the fitness world, we call this "eating clean," and to be able to compete, my diet had to be sparkling clean. Does that mean yours does too? Well, not completely, but the closer you get to clean and natural and the less processed stuff you have in your diet, the better and faster your results will be.

No Sugar, Please!

Eliminating foods with added sugar will help to prevent weight gain and promote quick and easy fat loss. Did you know that sugar literally acts like a drug in your system and can be compared to drug addiction? As long as it is in your diet, you will crave it. The more of it you eat, the more you will want, due to the physiological responses in the body. I found out the hard way that it takes two weeks to completely eliminate cravings related to sugar, once eliminated from your diet.

If I eat something that has a large amount of sugar in it, like birthday cake, it takes me two weeks before my cravings will go away again. This happens each and every time I choose to eat it, and what's worse is that the cravings will get stronger toward the end of those two weeks, right before they stop completely. This is how long it takes for this substance—and the drug-like effect—to get out of your system fully. I'll even crave alcohol toward the end of those two weeks as well, and I don't drink that often enough for me to even want it.

The reason for the alcohol craving is that it responds like sugar in your system and starts entering your bloodstream as soon as you take your first drink via immediate absorption in your mouth. Therefore, drinking alcohol can cause cravings too. Once you get past those first two weeks, you will find that your cravings go away completely. You'll even be able to sit there and watch someone eat junk right in front of you without having the urge to eat it yourself.

This is something I have noticed with myself, and when I educate my clients on this, they say it works the same for them as well. Cravings can be completely eliminated, as long as you keep the triggers mentioned in check. Each and every time you don't, you may notice that you're getting cravings again, and then all you have to do is use what you've learned to eliminate them again by making some simple tweaks to your diet.

STOP THE PATH OF DESTRUCTION (STARTING WITH WHAT YOU AND YOUR KIDS DRINK)

Sugary drinks alone, including soda and other carbonated beverages, are one of the main culprits for the declining health of our population as a whole. These substances should never be consumed as a main source of dietary fluids, but for many, it is the only thing they drink all day.

Meanwhile, they contain tons of empty calories, added sugars, food colorings, and caffeine. These ingredients have been shown in studies to cause liver damage, adrenal and thyroid burnout, bone loss, weight gain, and hyperactivity—all things that can lead to more dangerous diseases, like heart disease and diabetes. The caffeine and phosphoric acid alone cause calcium loss from the bones, weakening them over time.

Your body builds bone from the time you are born until approximately around age twenty-five; after that, you fight to maintain bone density or lose it. So imagine how weak your kids' bones will be if the process of building bones is interrupted because of carbonated beverages, especially those with caffeine.

We just might be seeing these same pop-drinking kids with osteoporosis by the age of forty or even younger. Did you know that for every twelve-ounce can of soda or carbonated beverage you drink you need one quart of water to rehydrate the body and one gallon of water just to correct the pH balance?

When your body's pH balance has been disturbed, it becomes fertile ground for disease and can cause weight gain or even prevent weight loss. Children learn from mirroring those around them, so if you are putting crappy, nutrient-absent junk food into your body, then your kids will too.

Remember what we've talked about throughout this book when it comes to changing your mind-set; what you do habitually and, in turn, what your children do habitually will affect both of you for the rest of your lives.

In other words, if you want to change the habits of your kids, then you will have to change your own habits first. In fact, when you lead by example, it is a win-win. Not only do you benefit from healthier choices, but so do your children!

I know it's difficult to make a change, especially one that not only affects you but your family and kids as well. I stopped drinking pop when I was about fifteen due to the negative effects it had on my health, so having pop in the house for my kids was never really a problem. I did, however, keep juice in the house. The initial changes I made included switching from drinks like Kool-Aid to real fruit juice and then from real fruit juice with added sugar to only the ones with no added sugars. Eventually I stopped keeping juice in the house altogether, and boy, when I made that decision, did my kids get upset. They complained for a good several months about the change but eventually got used to it. I figured if drinking water was a necessity for the human body and I was drinking it for those purposes, then why weren't my kids drinking it as well as their main source of liquid consumption?

It's good for their health too, and it will help to start a lifelong habit of drinking something that is good for them instead of something that's bad. It's always harder to make a lifestyle change well into your adult years, particularly when you've been practicing something day after day, week after week, year after year, for decades. Therefore, why not teach kids to eat healthy when they are young, thereby eliminating possible challenges before they start?

Interestingly enough, quite frequently these days my kids request water when we go out to eat or over to someone's house. Maybe not all the time, but a lot of the time. They still have juice or various soft drinks on occasion, but for the most part, water is the main source of fluid in their diets. The best part about it is that both of my kids have made comments years after the change about how they are glad that I made the change and taught them to drink water and eat healthy while they were young. They said that even though they may not have appreciated it at the time, they understand now how much better their lives are for it. Hearing that made up for all the complaining and begging that went on earlier when the initial changes were made. Best of all, I know that I have stopped a cycle of destruction and started a cycle of health within our family tree that will continue for generations to come.

STOP KILLING YOUR KIDS

For all of you parents out there, this message is for you: stop killing your kids. That's right, stop feeding them junk food. You know it is bad for you, and therefore you stay away from it, but then you go out and buy it for them. One of the biggest excuses people give me for bringing home unhealthy dietary choices is because their family members will not eat the healthy foods. Why?

Your family should be eating what you are eating. If it is good for you, it is good for them. Start your children off right by instilling lifelong healthy eating habits. Do you want them to be in your shoes when they are your age, struggling with their own weight? Of course not, so teach them while they are young and more receptive to it. The earlier you start creating healthy habits, the more likely it is to achieve lifelong weight-management success.

Remember when I said to surround yourself with healthy people? Well, why not start with your own family? Don't get me wrong; it is not going to be an easy task. It is definitely going to be more difficult to get your wife, husband, mother, or kids to eat carrots and drink water instead of candy bars and pop than for you to change your own habits. But with perseverance and dedication, you will not only create a healthy body for yourself, but you will develop a fit, focused lifestyle by creating a pro-active home environment.

With some slight alterations to your family's meal menu, everyone can be happy and healthy. As a matter of fact, get them involved. I let my kids choose any cereal they want from the shelf, as long as it is six grams of sugar or less. I taught them to read labels at age six. Why not? I love them and want them to be fit and healthy too. They will also help me plan healthy meals as well, which is great because I know they will eat them then.

The Third Fundamental:
Dietary Fiber

Intestinal health is a very important part of being healthy. In the alternative care world of health, it is often said that your blood is only as clean as your intestines. This means that if you're not eliminating properly, which should be after each meal, then your body can build up toxicity that can lead to many varying health problems.

Elimination rids your body of toxins and is a necessary part of maintaining your body's vitality on every level. There are lots of things in your diet that can prevent proper elimination, such as caffeine, low fiber intake, over-the-counter or prescribed medications, dehydration, and so on. Making sure you get an adequate amount of fiber in your diet can help you to maintain regular elimination of toxins, which, if left in the body, can eventually cause illness.

Dietary fiber is also a carbohydrate. Unlike other carbs, for the most part fiber is not used as a source of energy by your body; therefore, it does not add any extra calories to your plan. You need to consume at least twenty to thirty-five grams of fiber daily for maximum health benefits and proper elimination. Foods rich in fiber include fruits, vegetables, nuts, seeds, whole grains, and legumes (beans). There are a great many benefits related to getting the right amount of dietary fiber in your diet, and I have listed a few big ones below:

- Aids in weight loss because it prevents over-eating due to feelings of satisfaction after meals
- Regularity
- Lowered cholesterol levels
- Reduced risk of heart disease
- Reduced risk of hemorrhoids and/or lessens discomfort if you have them
- Prevention of colon cancer
- Protects against diverticulitis

Fiber is helpful in the control of blood sugar levels as well and can be an aid to decrease insulin requirements for those suffering from diabetes. If you are currently getting too little fiber in your diet, it is important to gradually increase fiber, while drinking an adequate amount of water as well. Gradually increasing fiber intake will allow your body to adjust, thus reducing intestinal distress and/or excessive gas production. Believe me on this one, you'll need to gradually increase the amount of fiber in your diet over time; otherwise, the intestinal distress and/or excess gas production will not be fun for you or people around you.

The Fourth Fundamental: *Vitamins*

Okay, we all know that vitamins are very important for building a healthy body. However, there are a few things that were surprising to me when I learned about them, so I thought I'd share a few things about vitamins with you that can be helpful in you reaching your goals. There are a total of thirteen vitamins that are needed by the body. They are divided into two groups: *water-soluble* and *fat-soluble*.

What this means is that water-soluble vitamins dissolve in water and are carried in the bloodstream. Vitamins can be found in a variety of foods, like fruits, vegetables, as well as whole grains, and the way you prepare those foods can have a large bearing on how much of those vitamins are available for your body. For instance, if you boil your veggies, they become nutrient deficient because vitamins are heat sensitive and become destroyed when boiled too long. Plus, some of the vitamins that dissolved in the water get strained into the drain with the water that they were boiled in. For maximum nutrient consumption, it is best to eat an abundance of raw foods, such as fruits and vegetables, so the vitamins are not destroyed by the heat.

Fat-soluble vitamins dissolve in fat. They are carried through your body attached to substances within your body that are made with fat. When your body utilizes the fat, it is then able to absorb the vitamins too. These types of vitamins are not lost during the cooking process, like water-soluble vitamins. Fat-soluble vitamins can be found in foods that contain fat, such as nuts, seeds, plant and fish oils, dairy products, and certain vegetables.

Fat-Soluble:

A	B2–Riboflavin
D	B3–Niacin
K	B6–Pyrodoxine
E	B12
	Folic Acid
	Panthothenic Acid
Water-Soluble:	Biotin
Tocopherol	Vitamin C–Ascorbic Acid
B1–Thiamin	

Vitamins play an important role in regulating a variety of bodily functions. They are essential for building bodily tissues, which include bones, skin, glands, nerves, and blood. Vitamins also assist in metabolism so that you are able to use energy from the foods you eat.

The three broad roles of vitamins are:

(1) Prevention of nutritional deficiencies
(2) Promotion of healing
(3) Produce and maintain overall good health

Vitamins are a crucial part of your daily diet, and it is suggested that you take a multivitamin/mineral supplement in an effort to receive all of your daily vitamin and mineral requirements for optimal health. As a trainer, I come across many individuals who begin taking individual vitamins, like A or C, after hearing about specific health benefits. Be sure to check with your doctor before doing this.

Excessive vitamin use is just as dangerous as vitamin deficiency. Vitamins can be taken in excess, resulting in toxicity and overdose. This usually only happens when a person takes several times what the RDA recommends via vitamin supplements, which is approximately eight times the daily suggested dosage. Did you know that it is nearly, if not completely impossible, to overdose on vitamins obtained through the foods you consume?

There are two more reasons to be careful when taking individual vitamins. The first reason is that they can cause adverse interactions in your body. As an example, I'll tell you about the time I started taking niacin due to some health benefits I had heard prior to learning about the dangers of taking lone vitamins. I remember that each time I would take it, within a short while, my entire body would become flush and red. I felt like I was burning up from the inside out. I read later that niacin can cause this type of flushing and that it is not necessarily a good thing, because too much niacin supplementation can cause liver damage. This is especially true if you are taking a prescribed medication from your doctor, which stresses the liver, and you then combine it with a lone vitamin, like niacin. You never really know what the results of this type of combination will cause; therefore, it's safer to take a multivitamin with the correct daily recommendations.

The second reason for choosing a multivitamin over lone vitamins is that certain vitamins facilitate the uptake of other vitamins, while some inhibit the absorption of others. For instance, vitamin C increases the absorption of iron, while calcium blocks the absorption of iron. Therefore, if you are taking extra calcium in your diet without the recommendation of your doctor, you may be hurting yourself rather than helping yourself. Multivitamin/mineral supplements have specific ratios of individual vitamins and minerals, which allows for maximum absorption of all vitamins and minerals.

You'll note this when you take a look at your multivitamin container and see that each vitamin has a different percentage of each individual nutrient per serving. Again, this is due to the supplement company creating a product that will allow for max absorption rates due to specific combinations and percentages of each individual nutrient.

When choosing a multivitamin supplement, keep in mind that tablets have fillers and binders, which are difficult for the body to break down. Because of this, you may not be able to absorb all of the nutrients from that tablet. Better choices include liquid, chewable, or capsule varieties to ensure maximum assimilation. Natural is usually a better choice over synthetic versions as well, because they are usually in a more available form for easy absorption by the body.

It is best to take your vitamins with a meal for maximum absorption and to prevent stomach upset. First thing in the morning or before bed are usually the best times to take them. There are a variety of brands out there, so do some research to find out more about the company and its reputation for distributing a good product. Nowadays the Internet is a great source for finding out more about what researchers find to be the best consumer product. Local health food stores or vitamin shops are another resource where you can ask about products to find the best one to suit your needs and budget.

The Fifth Fundamental: *Minerals*

The interesting thing about minerals is that they are often incorporated within the structures. For instance, the mineral calcium becomes a part of your bones and teeth, and when you don't get enough or you lose too much of this important nutrient, your bones and teeth can be weakened.

Some minerals also play an important role for maintaining your blood's pH balance. Blood pH must maintain 7.36 for optimal health. There are many chemical processes in the body that rely on this necessity. If it blood becomes too alkaline or too acidic, a number of complications can arise, including death. Eating lots of fresh foods that include a high amount of dark green, leafy vegetables has been getting some publicity these days due to the pH balancing effects they play on blood.

I'm big into "eating green," or eating a diet high in green vegetables, because I have seen amazing results both energetically as well as with maintaining a lean physique more easily. The results in my energy levels since I starting adding more fresh green vegetables in to my diet have been astounding. One of the reasons why eating green is so good for your body is due to the high mineral content in green vegetables, especially dark green, leafy ones.

There are fifteen different minerals that the body needs, which include calcium, chloride, chromium, copper, fluoride, iodine, iron, magnesium, manganese, molybdenum, phosphorus, potassium, selenium, sodium, and zinc. Other roles that minerals serve include providing structure in the formation of teeth and bones, maintaining normal heart rhythm, muscle contraction, nerve conduction, and the balance of bodily fluids, as well as playing an important role in cellular metabolism and serving as important parts of enzymes and hormones. Fresh one-ingredient foods are the best resources for obtaining mineral-rich foods, such as fruits, vegetables, whole grains, sardines with the bones, et cetera.

When it comes to minerals, like vitamins, it is recommended that you take a multivitamin/mineral supplement to ensure proper ratios for max absorption. If you are not eating six small meals a day, not eating all the recommended servings from each food group, and are not eating a large percentage of fresh foods in your overall meal plan, then you are most likely not getting all the nutrients your body needs. Therefore, almost everyone should take a multivitamin/mineral supplement as part of their regular nutritional regimen.

Taking a daily multivitamin/mineral supplement will help prevent deficiencies and create a healthier, more energetic you. If you cannot get in as much fresh foods as you like, then keep this in mind: fresh is best, frozen next, and canned as a last resort.

The Sixth Fundamental: *Fats*

Fats, like carbs, are a source of energy but in a more condensed form. This energy source supplies fatty acids, which are necessary for many of your body's activities. Two such fatty acids are linoleic and alpha-linoleic acid (omega-6 and 3 fatty acids). Both are essential fatty acids that must come from the food you eat. They are needed to make hormones and cell membranes and also ensure proper growth in children. Fats are usually referred to as "good" or "bad" fats because they each affect the body in different ways.

"Good" fats, or unsaturated fats, are needed for joint lubrication and for fat-soluble vitamin absorption. Plus, you need fat to burn fat. A diet too low in fat or fat-free can also lead to deficiencies of fat-soluble vitamins. The fat-soluble vitamins beta-carotene and vitamin E, along with the water-soluble vitamin C, are also known as antioxidants, and they prevent free radical damage in the body.

Free radicals are destructive cells that come from pollutants and toxins, which enter your body from the air you breathe, the food you eat, and can even be absorbed through your skin. Think of free radicals like a destructive cell that gets into your body and bounces around like a pinball in a pinball machine. The only problem is that everything it touches it destroys. Antioxidants adhere to these free radicals and prevent them from causing any damage. It is kind of like wrapping a destructive free radical cell with Bubble Wrap. Damage caused by free radicals is what causes old age and disease.

Unsaturated fats can appear on food labels as polyunsaturated or monounsaturated as well. They are liquid at room temperature and come from plant sources such as nuts, seeds, avocados, oils (canola, safflower, soybean, olive, peanut), and olives, as well as fish. The key to remember when it comes to fat is choosing foods that have antioxidant-rich unsaturated fats over those that have saturated unhealthy fats. Unsaturated fats also play in important role on your cholesterol levels. They help to lower LDL, or the bad cholesterol, while increasing HDL, or the good cholesterol. This positive effect helps to keep your circulatory system, including your heart, healthy.

"Bad" fats, or saturated fats, generally come from meats, dairy products, and tropical oils, like coconut or palm. Saturated fats are typically solid at room temperature and play a negative role in the body and on cholesterol levels. Eating a diet high in saturated fats can increase your cholesterol levels, especially LDL cholesterol, and can lead to plaque buildup and blockage in your arteries, increasing your risk for developing heart disease.

Probably the most important concept to remember about fat is that it is a very condensed form of calories. Eating even a small amount of it can equate to a lot of calories, and if you do not use them, they will be stored as fat on your body. For best fat-loss results and for a healthy diet, try to keep fat intake no higher than 20 to 30 percent of your total daily calories. The American Heart Association recommends that we consume less than 7 percent of our calories from saturated fat.

Choose foods naturally low in fat, like fruits, vegetables, and whole grains. Eat boneless, skinless chicken breast, turkey breast, and fish, instead of steak or fried foods. I know some of you reading this might be thinking, *But what about my wings?*

I'm not saying you can never have those types of foods again; what I am saying is that 90 percent of the time, eat for health, and 10 percent of the time, eat to cheat. By choosing naturally low-fat foods most of the time, you will reduce the total number of calories you eat, promoting weight loss, while preventing fat storage and weight gain. Because fat is a necessity for fat burning, when adding good fats to your diet, choose those from nuts, seeds, flax, and other unsaturated sources, such as olive oil or canola oil.

ecause you'll find that water is your
t comes to building and maintaining a
arned very early in my career that water
ortant nutrient in the body. In fact, your
body is composed of about 75 percent water. The nutrient is so vitally important that you will only be able to
survive approximately seventy-two hours without it.

Water is necessary for all of your body's systems to
run effectively and efficiently. Your body uses water for
digestion; circulation; temperature regulation; digestion
of carbs, proteins, and fats; and transportation of nutrients, such as minerals, vitamins, phytonutrients, and antioxidants, to your body's cells. Water also carries oxygen
through the bloodstream to all the tissues of the body. To
sum it up, water is involved with virtually every process
in the human body.

Studies have shown that not drinking enough water
results in dehydration and causes low energy levels,
fatigue, lack of concentration, depression, anxiety, joint
pain, cravings for sweet and/or salty foods, dizziness, dry
eyes, headaches, water retention, and even constipation.
Dehydration prevents the brain from getting enough
oxygen, which is the cause for many of these related
symptoms.

There are a number of other factors that cause dehydration, which include consuming dehydrating substances such as coffee, tea, soda pop, and salt. If you have
a job that requires you to talk a lot or travel via airplanes
frequently, it is also very easy for you to become dehy-

drated. Did you know that just talking can make you dehydrated if you do it enough and don't drink enough water? That's right; speaking entails exhaling while making sounds, and during the exhaling process, you release water in the form of mist.

Geography is another factor you must consider when it comes to maintaining hydration. Living in hot, dry climates causes increased water loss through sweat and low humidity levels in the air you breathe; therefore, it is imperative that you drink even more water in areas such as Arizona, Texas, California, and any other areas that have a dry climate.

A common excuse I frequently hear for individuals not drinking enough water is that they are just not thirsty. Thirst is a poor indicator for hydration because by the time you feel thirsty your body is already partially dehydrated. To prevent your body from becoming dehydrated, drink a minimum of eight to twelve eight-ounce glasses of water daily.

There are several easy ways to monitor your hydration levels. One easy way to tell if you are drinking enough water is by paying attention to your urination cycle: you should excrete two and a half to three quarts of water daily. An even easier method to determine hydration is to check the clarity of your urine. If your urine is yellow, frothy, or has a pungent smell, then you are dehydrated. Your urine should be clear or very close to it. There should also be little to no smell when your body is truly hydrated as well.

What about the discoloration you experience from taking vitamins? Vitamins will turn your urine yellow, but it is usually a very bright or florescent yellow color and usually occurs within a few hours of taking your vitamins. Try to recognize the difference between dehydration and vitamin discoloration so you know whether you are dehydrated or just eliminating excess vitamins that your body did not absorb.

Your eyes can be used as another assessment tool used for identifying dehydration. The symptoms vary, but if you pay close attention when you know that you have not had enough water, you will find that you may also experience one or more of these symptoms: dry, itchy, and/or red eyes. A heavy, watery feeling in your eyes can be another symptom. When your body is dehydrated, your eyes will start producing tears to keep the eyeballs moistened, and because tears have saline in them, it makes the eye feel heavier and more watery than usual.

Use your skin or complexion for monitoring this as well. When your face is oily, it usually means that you are not getting enough water. Take leather, for instance: it has to be conditioned; otherwise, it becomes dry and may even crack if it becomes too dry. Leather comes from the skin of animals, and just like leather, our skin needs to be conditioned. When you drink water and your body is hydrated, your skin is soft and supple, but when you become dehydrated, the glands in your face start producing oil to keep your skin from drying out. Other parts of the body may become dry too; you may notice this when other parts of your body become chalky and flaky.

When lacking in water, your feet, especially around the heels, become dry, hard, and may even appear to have deep cracks or crevices, similar to what you see in dirt after a drought.

Achy joints, muscle pain, and signs of arthritis can also be symptoms of dehydration. I have had many a client come to me over time that were experiencing what they thought was arthritis, which was the result of living in a state of perpetual dehydration. Once informed about these simple ways in which to monitor their fluid levels and then encouraged to alter their diets to accommodate more water intake, their symptoms went completely away.

Dehydration can produce a multitude of negative effects in the body, so be sure to monitor your fluid levels regularly and increase water intake as needed. Do you get that sluggish, tired feeling around three or four in the afternoon each day? Then you might be dehydrated. When this happens or you find it hard to concentrate during some part of your day, try drinking a glass of water to revive yourself. If you wait about twenty minutes, you'll usually find that doing this does the trick.

It's truly amazing all of the little signs your body gives off when it needs something. These are just a few of the signs I have discovered, with myself and from working with clients over the years, where the body is telling you exactly what it needs, but because no one has made it a point to let you know these things, these signs go unnoticed and chucked up as something they are not.

If you are currently not drinking water, then start by increasing your total water consumption slowly. Begin by drinking one quart a day, then increase by one-quart increments over the course of a four- to six-week period until you reach the desired goal of one gallon of water daily. Your body needs time to adjust; otherwise, if you start drinking too much too fast, you may notice a feeling of being waterlogged, where water sits in your stomach and swishes around because your body is not able to absorb it fast enough. An easy way to regulate your water intake is to get one-quart bottles and set a goal to drink one quart every three hours upon waking.

Setting a schedule works very well for accomplishing your hydration goals. A trick that helped me over the years was to create a simple schedule: if you are drinking four quarts a day, then try drinking quart one by 9:00 a.m., quart two by 12:00 p.m., quart three by 3:00 p.m., and your last quart by 6:00 p.m. This way, you achieve your goal without losing track.

This will allow you to become hydrated early in the day, when your body needs it most, and it will give you enough time before bedtime to ensure a restful sleep so you're not waking up during the night for frequent bathroom breaks. Oh, and get used to going to the bathroom every hour. Hourly bathroom breaks are a good thing because with every bathroom break you are excreting toxins out of your body, toxins that could otherwise cause sickness and disease.

IT'S ALIVE!

As I mentioned earlier, eating lots of mostly fresh, alive foods in your diet is the best thing you can do for your body, and you'll be amazed by the results when you do. Adhering to this tip caused my energy levels to go through the roof. Plus, my body stays much leaner more easily, and an effect I didn't expect was that my emotional and mental health was enhanced dramatically.

I feel less stressed on a regular basis, more calm all the time, yet full of energy and vitality like that which I had when I was a kid. And because my energy levels are higher, I have noticed that it's easier to stay disciplined with my diet and exercise routine, as well as other daily tasks. I hadn't realized until after making this change to my diet that when you feel tired and worn out all the time, it feels like it takes almost too much energy to eat right and exercise. I don't like admitting that, but it's true.

Even as a fitness professional that totally and completely believes in the value of eating right and exercising, I have gone through periods of time when it seemed too difficult to stay on track. I remember after competing for a couple of years that I felt something had changed. I used to feel energetic all the time, and for some reason, I had hit a brick wall and found it difficult to work out the way I used to.

I have always loved working out pretty intensely and always felt invigorated when I did, but after a couple years of competing, that had changed. I didn't feel energized after my workouts anymore. Instead, I felt like I needed to go home and go to bed. I felt dead, overworked, burned out, and found it extremely difficult to stay on track with my program. I started working extremely light just to make it through my workouts without feeling dead.

This feeling of being burned out went on for couple of years. I tried everything: drinking more water, taking various multivitamins, keeping my diet clean, changing up my workouts completely, and even taking a lot of extra time off of working out to let my body heal. I even began to think that maybe this was it; maybe everyone was right about what happens to your body as you age, that you have less and less energy over time until you finally become sedentary.

I'd argue with myself mentally, thinking, *No way, I just can't believe that to be true.* I know of people that have lots of energy and are in great shape well into the later years of their life. I have goals that I want to keep, and I won't give into that way of thinking. I want to be able to do the splits and a handstand when I'm, like, ninety years old! I just didn't want to give in and give up my goals or my way of life. Plus, feeling drained all the time just wasn't something I was willing to accept. I felt like I wasn't "me" anymore. Then I started to hear about eating green and how blood pH can affect your energy and vitality. I was intrigued and needed to learn more, and here's what I learned.

Eating mostly alive foods is of key importance, but when eating fresh foods, it is also important to incorporate lots of green vegetables into your meal plan. The truth is that when you are eating highly processed foods regularly, you may end up feeling like I did all the time as well, but when you eat fresh foods, the opposite is true. Highly processed foods are mostly, if not fully, dead and therefore cannot provide the vital alive energy you are looking for and that your body needs.

I believe this to be true for most people, because just about every American city has a coffee shop just about on every street corner. The problem is that coffee only provides you with superficial, life-draining energy that doesn't last. Once the coffee's caffeine kick wears off, you usually have even less energy than you did before you drank it. When you're emotionally and mentally exhausted, everything else seems to take too much effort. Since I started eating lots of fresh, alive foods and especially green veggies, that sort of exhaustion is a thing of the past.

Food that is picked fresh has the highest nutrient content and benefits for your body when compared to processed foods. Fresh food is alive and gives life to the body. Processed food is dead and can't provide the body with that same sort of vital life energy. Don't believe me? Try this little experiment: set a piece of highly processed white bread, along with an apple, on your kitchen table. What happens to the apple over time? What happens to the white bread? The apple rots and dies, while the white bread becomes stale and hard. The bread stays that way for who knows how long, until it turns to dust and blows away. The alive food dies, and the dead, processed food just sits there. This is true for all fresh foods and most processed foods.

The more processed a food is, the worse it is for your body, especially energetically. This is the number one reason why I encourage fresh foods as a top pick when it comes to attaining amazing overall health and vitality. Try it for yourself and see the difference.

STEP 4:

Meal Planning

Now that you understand the basic fundamentals regarding nutrition, the challenge becomes knowing what to do with the information. In other words, you need to know how to organize it in a way that works for you personally.

In the previous step, you learned how food affects your body and why it is important, but where do you start, and how do you put what you have learned into practice?

In this step, you'll learn how timing plays an important role in reaching your nutrition and fitness goals. You will also learn how to read food labels, understand recommended daily servings, serving sizes, and, finally, meal planning. Upon completion of this step, you will have a real grasp on what healthy eating entails from a fitness competitor's perspective and how you can create your own personalized plan, regardless of your health and fitness goals.

The recommendations in this step originate from a combination of several areas, the first being the USDA's MyPyramid guidelines, which can be found at www.mypyramid.gov. The tools on this site are designed for age appropriate nutritional needs, which will be helpful for families. Information in this section also includes the food strategies of athletes and fitness competitors, along with over eighteen years of client experience and personal life trial and error.

Many of the principles and most successful strategies that I learned and implemented into my own lifestyle over the years were those that came from fitness competitors. Therefore, some of the information I discuss here may sound slightly different from what you have heard before. However, if you take the time to talk to any fit individual that you know personally, a fitness competitor, or bodybuilder, you will most likely find that they adhere to many of the same dietary principles mentioned in this section. That is why they are in great shape, how they got there, and how you can get there too. You may not have the same goals in mind, and even if your dream isn't to compete, you can use the same strategies that have led to the success of those that make a living at looking good to help you with your personal goals.

NUTRITIONAL GUIDELINES

The first step in food planning begins with the USDA's MyPyramid. The USDA (United States Department of Agriculture) has created guidelines regarding food consumption so Americans can make better nutritional decisions for improving their health. You can find MyPyramid with the RDA (Recommended Daily Allowances) for each of the various food groups, including grains, vegetables, fruits, milk, meat and beans, oils, and discretionary calories, by visiting www.mypyramid.gov.

Changes that were made to the food pyramid in recent years include the addition of suggested activity levels. The daily nutritional recommendations are based on an individual's age, gender, and amount of exercise or activity they participate in daily.

When devising a personalized food plan, there are other aspects of a well-balanced program that you should understand. One of these aspects includes the developmental stages that your body undergoes and its nutritional needs during those times.

When making good dietary choices, it is important to keep in mind your personal fitness goals as well as the nutritional needs of the body during different stages of development. This will allow you to make better-informed decisions, which will complement these stages of growth, while fulfilling your basic food-based needs along the way.

Dietary needs vary depending upon which developmental stage of growth the body is undertaking. There are three major stages of growth, and during those stages, your body requires a large percentage of its caloric needs from a specific macronutrient base. Let's take a look at the needs of those three major stages of development so you have a better understanding of how your body necessitates changes in meal structure and macronutrient needs at different ages in your life.

THE FIRST MAJOR STAGE
OF DEVELOPMENT

The first stage covers birth to two years of age. The macronutrient needs for this stage of development require that fat is the largest percentage of macronutrient needed by the body, followed by protein, and finally carbohydrates.

During this stage, the human body is growing at such a fast pace that caloric needs are extremely high when comparing the caloric needs at other stages and taking into consideration body size. In fact, by the end of the first year of life, a baby has already tripled its birth weight. Boys around four years of age are already 59 percent of their total adult height and girls are 64 percent of theirs.

That is amazing! You are more than halfway grown by the time you reach only four years of age. Due to this amazing rate of growth, babies require a very high percentage of fat in their diets. Fat is not the only macronutrient infants and toddlers require, but it is the most predominant nutrient needed for proper brain development and physical growth. In fact, 60 percent of the brain, plus the sheaths that encapsulate nerves, is made up primarily of fat. In addition, due to the tiny size of a baby's stomach, they need nutrient-dense foods to ensure proper caloric needs are being met for such an exponential growth rate.

THE SECOND MAJOR STAGE
OF DEVELOPMENT

Between the ages of two and six, the percentage of fat and carbohydrate needs for a child slowly adjusts, reflecting a need for less fat and more carbohydrates. At this stage, the human body is experiencing continued growth; therefore, energy foods consume a high percentage of a person's diet for the proper development of organs, bones, muscles, tendons, ligaments, hormones, et cetera. Plus, this is a time in life during which activity is high and where playtime and sports may take up a large portion of the day.

Around the time of puberty, when major changes in lifestyle may occur, energy requirements begin to change once again. The development of organs, bones, muscle, tendons, ligaments, hormones, et cetera, continues during this stage, but lifestyle changes play a role in the amount of some of those needs. These changes vary from person to person, because some kids may continue to play organized sports well into their young adult years while others discontinue and lead a more sedentary lifestyle. Those involved in organized sports will have higher caloric expenditures as a result and usually require a larger amount of carbohydrates in response. Either way, carbohydrates continue to consume a high percentage of one's diet during these stages of development because your body can have continued growth up until around age twenty-five.

A major reason why many individuals begin gaining excess fat or weight after this watershed age is due to lessening caloric needs in response to the discontinuation of growth. When compacted with significant lifestyle changes, weight can become a real problem for the first time for some after the age of twenty-five because of those alterations.

Tastes Like Teen Spirit

The most prevalent problem regarding the diets of children and teens today is that they are eating the wrong types of foods, especially the wrong types of carbohydrates. Instead of consuming mostly whole grains, they are choosing highly processed, preprepared packaged products that have loads of added sugar, fats, and artificial additives.

Whereas health professionals and *Dietary Guidelines for Americans* suggest very few sweets, modern teenagers are eating vast amounts of them and drinking sugar-laden beverages such as pop, sport drinks with added caffeine, and juices with tons of added sugars and artificial additives. Some of those additives actually increase appetites and cravings, which, in many cases, lead to overweight and obesity. In fact, the New York Department of Mental Health and Hygiene and the Department of Education found that one out of every four children is overweight or obese.

Overweight kids? I mean, what is going on here? Well, just take a look at their lunch menus; there usually are not many healthy choices on there. Even though schools are offering healthier menu options, there are a lot of unhealthy foods available as well.

The problem that occurs is that a high percentage of kids will choose what tastes good over what is healthy for them. An average school's lunch menu may consist of pizza, milk (white and chocolate), French fries, burgers on processed white buns, and some sort of fruit, usually packed in high sugary syrup. Yummy, just what every kid loves (but not necessarily what they need, nutritionally speaking).

There have been several changes over the last few years in relation to the Bush administration's goals of decreasing and preventing youth obesity rates, but many of the unhealthy choices continue to be available as well, and again, many kids will usually go for unhealthier choices over healthier ones.

Healthy choices do not have a chance in many cases, especially since processed foods have additives that enhance flavors and produce cravings, due to the physiological effects of those additives. What about the whole grains, lean proteins, fresh vegetables without salt and butter and no sugar added, or just plain fresh fruit choices? Thanks to modern technology and their attraction to hungry teenagers, fresh, unprocessed, "clean" foods barely stand a chance.

Whatever happened to good, old-fashioned water?

It is, after all, what the body needs. Unfortunately, children are not getting what the *Dietary Guidelines for Americans* recommends nutritionally, due to the prevalent unhealthy products so widely available to kids in the market today. Instead, they are getting a diet that poorly nourishes the body, promotes body fat, creates fertile ground for disease, and inhibits concentration, therefore negatively affecting learning propensity.

Many health-related problems that were once seen mainly in adults, such as high cholesterol, hyperactivity, overweight and obesity, depression, anxiety, and type 2 diabetes (once termed adult-onset diabetes), are now becoming more pervasive in younger populations. The negative health trends affecting the younger population are the direct result of poor nutritional standards practiced by kids and young adults today.

THE THIRD MAJOR STAGE OF DEVELOPMENT

The next stage of development encompasses ages twenty-five and up. As an adult, you are not really growing anymore unless, unfortunately, it's in the width department. Instead, you are maintaining the life of your cells and repairing bodily tissues. You do not have the same energy needs you once did when you were younger; therefore, you shouldn't be eating the same way you ate during the other stages of growth.

As explained, the lifestyle and activity of most adults changes drastically after childhood. For many, daily routines evolved from playing all day long to sitting for the majority of the day instead. Calorie expenditure has changed considerably in response to decreases in activity levels; therefore, your body does not need as many high-energy foods as it once did, such as fat and carbohydrates. That means eating ice cream in front of the TV may not be the best choice when your calorie needs have changed as an adult. Though you may desire these types of foods, unfortunately in most cases, it's not something your body needs. Your body needs food that promotes health and tissue repair. After age twenty-five, your body spends most of its energy healing and detoxifying. Consequently, it's important that you consume dietary choices that will provide the necessary nutrients for expediting these processes.

Some of the foods that promote healing and cleansing benefits are proteins, fruits, vegetables, and water. Carbohydrate requirements decrease drastically as we age and as our lifestyles evolve.

Grains remain an important food group that should be included in a well-rounded nutritional plan, but due to lowered caloric needs, lower calorie vegetables are a great alternative to some of those higher calorie carbohydrates you're used to eating, as a way to lower and maintain your weight. Adding vegetables to your diet can be very helpful when it comes to attaining and keeping your body lean. They are packed with nutrients, they are alive, and they are usually low in calories, making them a great alternative when it comes to lessening the amount of calories in your diet.

Athletes, at any age, have a higher carbohydrate need than nonathletes do; therefore, it is important to take this into consideration when developing your own personal meal plan. Play around with the amount and kinds of carbohydrates in your diet. You may first want to try replacing highly processed carbohydrates with whole grain selections. Next, you can begin lessening the total amount in your diet by replacing them with lower calorie veggies. After making these adjustments, wait a few weeks to see how your body responds. It is common to find that with each alteration to your diet and exercise program, your body gets leaner each time.

THE FITNESS INDUSTRY MAKES ITS OWN RULES

When referring to the fitness industry, what I am essentially referring to is the competitive fitness arena. Over the years I had taken classes and studied what the dietetic world promoted as a balanced and health orientated diet, but to tell you the truth, even though I practiced those principles in my meal planning, I never got the results I was truly looking for.

Once I decided competing was in my future, I started picking the brains of other competitors to find out what I was doing wrong. The problem was not that I was doing something wrong; the problem was that the actions I was partaking in were results-driven based on the dietetic arena and USDA's standards and vision of health. In other words, their goals and mine were not aligned; therefore, I had to find what actions would align with my personal fitness goals. Eventually I found that connection in the world of competitive fitness. Like a lot of people, my goals started with appearance rather than health, but over time, I found the two go hand in hand, and the alterations I made to my diet produced amazing results in both areas.

My original intentions focused on my personal appearance, which was to look like I was fit. Health has a "look," and that look is what I wanted. In order to reach that goal, I sought out the advice and recommendations of other fit-looking people, which included fitness competitors. What I found was that these people had a different set of rules they lived by to create purpose-driven results.

Some of those rules were very different from what I had previously learned and even what the USDA and medical world promoted. I took a leap of faith and started implementing them one by one. I only focused on one at a time so that I could master it. Mastering it meant that it had then become a habit, which only needed to be maintained. Habits are hard to break, good or bad.

The only reason people are out of shape or not reaching their personal fitness goals is because they have habits that are not producing the results they want, so in a sense, they are "bad" habits. If you are not getting the results you want, then the habits and behaviors you are practicing need to be changed until they start producing the results you *do* want.

I did not change everything all at once. Instead, I changed one thing at a time, and sometimes those changes took a while to master, but now I practice those habits each and every day without even thinking about them, and the results I have gotten are a direct result of implementing what I learned from others.

The fitness industry makes its own rules when it comes to dietary guidelines, and I am going to give you those rules. The rules that competitors live by are outcome-driven in nature and geared toward producing a lean physique.

By implementing these rules into your daily nutritional choices and lifestyle, you will create an internal physiological balance, as well as a toned body, and this internal balance will enhance your outward appearance, along with true energy and vitality. Your body will have the necessary nutrients to heal itself of injury, as well as provide the building blocks necessary for constructing the body you have always wanted and deserve.

- Rule One: *Eat Clean*
- Rule Two: *Drink One Gallon of Water Daily*
- Rule Three: *Say "No" to the Three S's (Sugar, Salt, and Sauces)*
- Rule Four: *Correspond Food Choices with Time of Day*
- Rule Five: *Eat Every Three Hours*
- Rule Six: *No Dairy*
- Rule Seven: *Consume Little to No Alcohol*
- Rule Eight: *Consume Three to Four Servings of Protein throughout the Day*
- Rule Nine: *Rotate Your Calories*

Rule One: *Eat Clean*

Rule number one is to eat clean, but what does this mean exactly? This concept goes back to eating one-ingredient fresh foods that leave little to no toxic waste in the body. Toxins that come from added ingredients in food are what clog up our system and prevent organs from working to their fullest potential.

Think of it this way: if you put dirty oil in your car, the motor is not protected and lubricated properly, and small bits of dirt can actually destroy working parts, increasing friction, heat, and therefore break down the engine and its working parts more quickly. As you know, if the motor does not work, then you either have to replace the engine or the entire car itself.

On the other hand, if you replace necessary fluids and you change its oil every three thousand miles, then the engine remains in good working condition, with only a few minor maintenance issues coming up from time to time. Nowadays, engines can last up to two hundred thousand miles, and just like your car engine, your body can last a long time too. That is *if* you take care of it by putting in "clean" foods instead of junk foods that only clog the system and destroy its working parts.

Fitness competitors eat to build their body to a specific state. That is, they eat for nutritional benefit, which is an outcome-driven result. Unfit people may eat for other reasons, like addiction or emotional pleasure. To change your mind-set, you must first determine what is more important to you: quick, physical pleasure or long-term health. Food is a necessity the body has to have for fuel, growth, and healing, not emotional drowning.

As mentioned earlier, additives in foods also create cravings and cause overeating. Eating clean does not produce these same effects. Think about it: when was the last time you overate on apples or Brussels sprouts? Probably never, right? And why do you think that is? It is because there are not any additives that make you crave more.

When you crave natural foods, it is usually due to your body needing some nutrient from that food, and once you have gotten enough of the nutrient your body needs, your craving goes away. For instance, you may crave carrots because your body needs beta-carotene. But when you crave processed foods, it is the additives that you are craving, and those additives can be addictive in nature, so the more you eat, the more your body will want and the more you will crave that food. So clean, unprocessed food should be the main staple in your diet so that your body gets what it needs.

Rule Two: *Drink One Gallon of Water Daily*

A common concept in fitness circles is that drinking water leads to weight loss for a variety of reasons. Want to burn some extra calories effortlessly and do something good for yourself? Then try drinking one gallon of cold water a day. If the water temperature is colder than your body temperature, it cools down your core temperature;

therefore, your body has to work on getting it back up to 98.6 degrees.

Did you know you could burn an extra five hundred calories a day *just* by drinking cold water? Jogging on the treadmill for an hour at four miles per hour may not even burn that many calories, so start drinking more water today and increase the speed at which you reach your personal fat-loss goals. If you don't like cold water, that's okay; drinking room temperature water causes you to burn calories too.

Consuming water is like drinking negative calories because your body has to metabolize it, and there aren't any calories in it for you to have to burn later. The fitness industry has known this for a long time, and it is the number one reason why you see fit people drinking water and not soft drinks or other processed fluids. Try eliminating dehydrating beverages like coffee and pop from your diet as well because the negative side effects can cause your metabolism to run sluggish.

Actually, for every eight- to twelve-ounce cup of coffee you drink, your body will excrete as much as a quart of water, due to coffee's diuretic effects. Therefore, you will need an additional quart of water to rehydrate for every cup of coffee you drink. For every single can of pop you drink, you'll need one gallon of water just to bring your body back to its normal pH balance. Therefore, to answer a common question regarding counting the coffee, tea (black and brown), pop, flavored waters, carbonated drinks, and most other liquids toward your water intake, the answer is *no!*

Water is water and precisely what your body requires for optimal health. You would not put olive oil in your engine in place of car oil, would you? Of course not. Even though they may both possess a few similar properties, they are different substances entirely. One will keep your car running efficiently, and the other will destroy the engine. Water goes in clear and comes out clear. Coffee, brown and black tea, pop, and other liquids go in brown or some other color and come out yellow. Where does the color go?

Most of those colorings and chemicals stay in the body and can build up over time. Toxic buildup over years prevents your organs and cells from functioning properly and can cause cellular mutation. This cellular mutation is how cancer gets its start. The same cells that used to keep your body healthy are what could eventually kill you over time, due to toxicity from ingredients you consume in your daily diet that your body does not need or want. The more toxic the food is that you eat, the more toxic your body becomes and the higher your risk is for developing cancer and other diseases.

Be wary of the negative effects on the body when it comes to consuming caffeinated beverages. There are many beverages on the market today that have added caffeine, which can negatively affect any health conditions that you may already have, such as high cholesterol, diabetes, high blood pressure, and so on.

Caffeinated beverages can also play a negative role when it comes to weight gain and loss as well. Since caffeine is a nervous system stimulant, it is a common conception that it aids in fat metabolism and weight loss. Due to its diuretic effects, however, it dehydrates your body, therefore creating water loss instead of fat loss. This dehydrating effect can lead to cravings, as mentioned earlier.

The stimulating effects of caffeine can also lead to increased stress levels, which stimulate the productions of hormones like cortisol. It has been documented that such increases in these types of hormones lead to increased appetite and the deposit of excess abdominal fat as well. Therefore, drinking caffeinated beverages can actually be preventing you from reaching your weight loss goals or dreams of having a flat tummy. Contrary to popular belief, coffee and other caffeinated beverages, such as energy drinks like Red Bull, do not give you energy. Instead, they steal your existing energy by causing you to burn it faster than you normally would. The effects of consuming stimulants like caffeine will leave you feeling sluggish, tired, stressed, lethargic, depressed, anxious, and overworked.

The toxic effects of caffeine also build up in your system and can lead to achy joints, weakened muscle tissue, decreases in bone density, raised blood pressure, and lowered immune system. Eliminating caffeine can be challenging because it is an addictive substance and the removal of it from your diet can cause headaches, irritability, and, initially, low energy levels. Give yourself at least three days to get over the addiction part of it, about a week for headaches to subside, and a month for your energy levels to return to full, normal capacity.

Due to withdrawal symptoms, you may find it necessary to slowly eliminate caffeinated beverages, rather than eliminating them altogether. Try cutting your consumption down by anywhere from 25 to 50 percent every few weeks until completely eliminated. Once it is completely out of your system, you will find that you have an abundance of energy; your vitality will be much higher in a month's time than it ever was while drinking coffee. Client after client has thanked me repeatedly for educating them about the negative effects of stimulants because of how amazing they feel after eliminating it from their diet completely.

In summary, water is what the body needs, and anything else can be preventing your weight loss success. Even if you do not initially like drinking water, keep practicing this proactive habit. You will be surprised how after a while your body will begin to crave it.

Try this suggestion to help you accomplish your goal of drinking a gallon a day: keep a water bottle with you wherever you go; keep bottles of water at your desk, in your car, in your purse, and around the house. You will find that if it is sitting there you will naturally reach for it and take a drink. In no time at all you will find that you are drinking more and more water and actually enjoying doing so. Your energy levels will be drastically increased, due to cellular hydration and thinner blood. When your body is hydrated, your blood is thinner and can travel throughout your body more easily. The easier it can move around, the less work your heart has to do. Plus, if your blood is circulating faster, then vital nutrients are getting to all of your cells more efficiently, keeping them alive and allowing them to get rid of waste faster.

Remember that vitamins and minerals can aid in weight loss, so if your blood is circulating faster, then your body is receiving those nutrients more quickly. Once again, keep water bottles everywhere, and you will find that eventually you feel lost if you do not have one in your hand.

Rule Three: *Say "No" to the 3 S's (Sugar, Salt, and Sauces)*

The only place I have ever heard this rule is in the competitive arena, and it is probably one of the toughest rules to implement and stick to. Like all habits, however, once you get in the groove of making sure these substances are eliminated from your diet, you will find it is an easy rule to maintain and well worth the effort.

SUGAR

Processed sugars that are added to food are the most disadvantageous substance anyone can consume, and it is the number one product that sabotages weight-management success.

Obesity trends have been on the rise throughout history due to the inventions of man, which have made life easier and reduced the amount of human labor needed. The increase in obesity and overweight had been steady over time until around the 1970s, when high-fructose corn syrup was introduced into the market. Since this introduction, obesity and overweight have skyrocketed almost overnight.

High-fructose corn syrup, corn syrup, corn syrup solids, and other similar products are the atomic bomb of energy or, in other words, an intensely condensed form of sugar that your body finds incredibly difficult to burn. It is just too much energy for your body to burn, plus it also has negative effects on the body in a variety of other ways. I have heard from alternative or complimentary care physicians that processed sugars can increase pain throughout the body due to the inflammatory effects they cause. It fluctuates blood sugar levels and causes craving cycles. It also stresses the liver. In the *Super Size Me* documentary, professionals discuss a study done with children where their livers were biopsied to determine the effects of high-fructose corn syrup on the liver, and what they found was early signs of what could or even would eventually become cirrhosis of the liver.

In other words, these kids were developing a disease of the liver that normally is prevalent in alcoholics, but they were not drinking alcohol. Instead, they were eating large amounts of processed sugars in their diet, mainly in the form of high-fructose corn syrup. In the movie, we also see Morgan Spurlock's cholesterol levels and liver function skyrocket as well, which, according to the documentary, is a direct result of the high sugar content in the foods he was consuming.

Sugar destroys the body in a variety of ways, so eliminating added sugars will only enhance your results. Added sugar and natural fruit sugars are two completely different things. Sugar naturally present in food affects the body differently than processed sugars that are added to foods. When reading food labels, look to see if the sugar present in the food is naturally occurring, such as when there is fruit in the product, or if it was added. You'll be able to find out if sugar was added by looking at the ingredients. Some sugar additives to look for that will slow weight loss success and may even prevent it include brown sugar, corn sweetener, dextrose, maltodextrin, fructose, glucose, maltose, lactose, high-fructose corn syrup, corn syrup, corn syrup solids, malt syrup, raw sugar, and sugar. Foods that tend to be high in added sugars are soft drinks, candy, bakery items, a variety of alcoholic drinks, some sauces, ice cream, and other junk food treats.

SALT

Although salt is a necessary nutrient in your diet, most people are consuming entirely too much. Processed and prepackaged foods account for the highest percentage of sodium consumed in most people's diet.

Some foods, like smoked salmon, can contain almost 50 percent of your daily recommended dosage of sodium in one serving. The problem that arises with salt is if you are consuming too much your body can easily become dehydrated. The initial response that you will sometimes notice is that salt pulls water into the body, which accounts for that bloated feeling you get after eating a meal high in sodium.

Water accompanies the salt when leaving the body, thereby leaving your cells in a dehydrated state. As mentioned earlier, dehydration can lead to an array of negative effects, which ultimately can sabotage your weight loss efforts. Therefore, try to limit excess sodium intake, which usually occurs from consuming preprepared food or snack items such as frozen meals, canned items, soups, pretzels, nuts, chips, and other salted items. The USDA recommends limiting your salt intake to less than one teaspoon or 2,300 mg daily.

SAUCES

Though sauces add kick to any meal, they can also slow and even prevent progress toward your goals. Many sauces are comprised of a combination of added salts and sugars; both are added ingredients that fitness competitors try to minimize or eliminate in order to get lean.

Sauces tend to add additional unnecessary calories to your diet, which, if not burned, end up getting stored as fat. Those calories are usually in the form of fats and sugars, which make losing weight, getting fit, and becoming more lean more of a challenge for you.

The key is to eat those foods that will aid you in your efforts of becoming healthier, not interfere with them. "Less is best" when it comes to adding ingredients to the meals you consume, especially when those ingredients include large amounts of sodium, sugar, fats, highly processed carbs, and/or calories, as is the case with most sauces today.

Don't get me wrong; it is possible to find some sauces or toppings that are healthier, which may be lower in salt and sugar. But keep in mind the more extras you add to your meal, the more calories you'll have to burn later. And if you don't burn them you'll store them, adding more to what you already have, slowing your progress even more.

When I was growing up, there was a commercial on Saturday mornings that had a catchy tune that said, "Don't drown your food." Whenever I think of that commercial, I also sing the theme song in my head. So if I could send you on your way with one visual or audio message for this rule, it would be that one!

Rule Four: *Correspond Food Choices with Time of Day*

Your body has natural, oscillating rhythms referred to as *circadian rhythms.* These rhythms change like the rhythmic flow of waves washing upon the shore, moving in and out in a fluctuating pattern, which functions in correlation with your internal clock.

All of the body's functions, such as eating, sleeping, and detoxifying, are on this daily twenty-four-hour cycle and directly correspond with your metabolism. Understanding common functions of the body that occur during different segments of the day will be helpful in your efforts to get lean.

This information will give you a more in-depth understanding of how you can use food in accordance with the changes your metabolism goes through throughout the day. Consuming foods that support and work naturally with the various processes and fluctuations in metabolism will help you make better food choices.

Why bother? The effects of choosing foods that align with these fluctuations are maximized fat loss, lessened fat storage, and enhanced nutrient support the body needs for completing such processes like detoxification. Your body goes through various processes during the day, which are generalized in the list below:

- *First eight hours upon waking:* Active—hydrate and fuel
- *Second eight hours:* Less active—energy maintenance to decreasing metabolic rate
- *Third eight hours:* Rest—recover and healing

The major role of each of the three macronutrients—fat, protein, and carbohydrates—should correspond to your body's nutritional needs during these three segments of time listed above. Carbohydrates fuel and hydrate the body and include fruits, whole grains, beans, and vegetables. Fat lubricates the joints and also provides fuel and encompasses such foods as nuts, flaxseeds, and oils. Lastly, protein is the main staple your body needs for healing and tissue repair, which includes lean meats, eggs, poultry, fish, and high-quality protein supplements.

Upon waking each morning, your body is ready to eliminate the waste it has been removing during the healing and detoxification process throughout the evening; hence, the first thing you do is go to the bathroom upon waking. Because you have been sleeping for a number of hours without food or drink, your body is depleted and needs to be rehydrated and refueled for the day. Drinking plenty of water and eating foods that pull water into your cells is what your body requires most during this time. The best foods for expediting the fulfillment of these needs are fruits, whole grains, and other complex carbohydrates.

During the second stage of the day, your body becomes less active, especially toward the evening, so your metabolism begins naturally slowing down. Changes in metabolism occur in preparation for rest the closer you get toward bedtime. During this segment of the day, it is best to consume foods that promote healing and detoxification, which includes lean sources of protein and vegetables.

These food sources give your body the necessary macronutrients for carrying out these functions while you sleep. Eating in the evenings is not necessarily a bad thing; it is only counterproductive if you are eating the wrong types of foods, like complex carbohydrates, processed foods, and/or high-fat foods that your body will not have time to burn off before you go to bed. If you eat lean protein and veggies in the evening, your body will use them throughout the night instead of storing them.

Rule Five: *Eat Every Three Hours*

If you have children of your own or know someone that has children, you are probably familiar with the fact that babies eat approximately every three hours. This is no accident. That's because three hours is the natural metabolic cycle that your body runs on. Before I became aware of this concept, I was under the impression that if I wanted to burn fat I needed to eat less throughout the day. Therefore, I would starve myself by eating only one time a day.

Unfortunately, I never got the lean-looking body I was trying to attain by eating this way. I could always pinch an inch or more, even when I was starving myself. Then I found out that for maximum fat burning results, you need to eat small amounts of food every three hours, anywhere from four to six times a day. In other words, it's better to graze than to eat large meals.

Your body works on three-hour intervals, so if you eat more than what your body needs for fuel in the next three hours, the excess will be stored as fat. Only give your body just enough because each time you walk away from a meal feeling full, you are storing fat. Instead, leave a meal feeling content, not hungry nor full. Think of it like this: you cannot fill up the gas tank of your car for an entire month in one stop. If you tried, the excess gasoline would overflow. Only eat enough calories for the three hours of post-meal activity. This way, your tank gets a chance to be emptied out before the next meal, therefore preventing overeating and excess fat storage.

Skipping meals causes muscle breakdown, which slows metabolism. The key to building a lean physique is giving your body just enough, in frequent three-hour bouts, to prevent these negative changes in metabolism.

This will ensure that your body does not break down muscle, slowing metabolism. Instead, metabolism will remain high, and fat will be more easily burned, instead of stored over time.

Did you know that your stomach is only the size of your fist? Makes you wonder how you can fit so much more than a fist-size of a meal into it. Your stomach stretches and has the ability to shrink over time as well. When eating frequently throughout the day, it is important to eat smaller meals, keeping in mind that your stomach is the size of your fist. Eat fist-size amounts of food for snacks and meals. Try using smaller plates so you are not tempted to eat more than what your body needs. If you feel like you want to take a second helping, wait twenty minutes to be sure that you really feel hungry and it is not just low blood sugar making you think you want more. If you wait twenty minutes, your body will have broken down some of the food you ate, and your blood sugar levels will be more normal. In most cases, your first helping is all you need to feel satisfied, not that second helping.

When you make adjustments to your meal planning and lessen the amount of food you eat at one meal or snack, initially you may feel as though you are not getting enough and that your stomach is still empty. Your stomach will shrink back to normal after a few weeks, and these feelings will subside, creating a feeling of contentment after meals. You may make slight adjustments to your meal size over time, especially if you are used to eating larger portion sizes.

When first introducing more meals throughout the day, you may not feel hungry every three hours. The reason for this is that your metabolism is used to kicking in each day around the same time you normally eat because it has been trained to do so. If you eat at the same time every day, your body anticipates the future meal and starts preparing ahead of time by jump-starting your metabolism. If you begin to eat in three-hour intervals each day, your body will adjust over time by keeping the metabolism going during digestion and then maintaining it for the next incoming meal.

Like all good habits, give yourself time to adjust. After all, it takes about two weeks to start feeling the effects of this modification. After about two weeks, however, you will begin to feel hungry around every three hours because your metabolism is preparing for the incoming food. After about six weeks of implementing this new behavior, you will have established a new proactive and healthy habit that creates a faster metabolism and, as a result, produces successful fat loss.

Rule Six: *No Dairy*

Out of all the rules I learned during my competitive days, this one was the most surprising rule of all. Prior to learning this rule, I had a thorough understanding of how important protein was for building the body I wanted. Therefore, a large percentage of my protein needs came from the dairy group in the form of cheese, yogurt, ice cream, and milk.

After talking with several competitors and trainers, however, I came to realize that dairy had to go.

What a challenge this was going to be for me, since I would drink a glass of milk each night with my dinner and use it to make protein drinks as well. Once I got rid of dairy, or at least ice cream, milk, cheese, and yogurt, I was amazed at the results. People in fitness would talk about how dairy bloats your body and boy, does it ever. I lost five pounds in the first week of eliminating it, plus I felt better and looked leaner.

The best way to determine whether or not something in your diet has a negative effect on your fitness goals is to follow this simple four-step process:

(1) Eliminate the item for six weeks. So, for instance, if you're thinking of not doing dairy anymore—or even caffeine or some of the other nutritional changes we've discussed here—don't just skip it for a day or two and try to feel the effects; give yourself a full six weeks.

(2) Note how your body responds to the change in diet. Pay attention to your body during these six weeks, and consciously take time to note how you feel. In the case of caffeine, for instance, notice when your energy is lagging and when it picks up; try to tell if, after two weeks, then three, four, five, and six you can actually note the differences. Same with dairy; stop regularly during this time to physically and mentally cal-

culate whether or not you feel better or worse without the item.

(3) Reintroduce it. To tell if eliminating something from your diet is really having a positive or negative effect, after six weeks, reintroduce it to your diet.

(4) Note the change once again after it has been reintroduced. By giving yourself six weeks, you can really tell the difference in how something tastes, feels, or even affects your body. For instance, if you've been without caffeine for six weeks and suddenly drink a whole can of soda—wow, look out! You can immediately feel the jolt, and chances are it won't be as pleasant as the regularly balanced feeling of energy you get going caffeine-free. Likewise, with dairy, immediately after eating dairy after being off of it for six weeks, you will probably note how heavy, rich, and indulgent it feels—probably unpleasantly so.

Prior to the elimination of dairy, I was able to keep my weight down, but I was never able to accomplish that lean, toned look you see that's so prevalent in the fitness magazines. Once dairy was taken out of my diet, I discovered how easy it was to not only attain that look that I wanted but to maintain it easily as well.

Dairy produces a lot of negative side effects, especially for those wanting to reduce body fat. These side effects may go unnoticed until you eliminate diary and products containing dairy from your diet. When any sort of dairy is consumed, it causes immediate bloating and takes almost two days for this bloating to go completely away and for your body to return to its normal water balance. The lactose, which is a form of milk sugar, is the main precursor to these effects.

Everyone is basically lactose intolerant to some degree, but most of us are completely unaware of it. The reason for this intolerance is related to a decline in the enzyme lactase, which breaks down lactose in milk. This enzyme is highest at birth but declines at a relatively fast rate, decreasing approximately 95 percent between the ages of three and a half to five, and continues to decline with age.

Therefore, breaking down this nutrient found in milk becomes a very difficult process for the body. Due to this decline, which creates the inability to break down lactose, a process called "lactose malabsorption" results. The unabsorbed milk sugar then draws water into the bowel, which creates negative symptoms of bloating, flatulence, and cramping to some degree or another.

What about calcium? There are a variety of other calcium-rich foods, other than dairy, that will enable you to receive enough in your diet for bone health, such as:

- Broccoli
- Watercress
- Kale
- Okra
- Red kidney beans
- Chick peas

- Green beans
- Baked beans
- Almonds
- Brazil nuts
- Hazelnuts
- Sesame seeds
- Walnuts
- Tahini paste
- Sardines
- Whitebait fish
- Salmon
- Apricots
- Figs
- Currants
- Oranges
- Tofu
- Bok choy
- Turnip greens
- Fortified orange juice

In fact, dairy is acidic in your body, and when foods are acidic, your body needs to neutralize it in order to maintain a blood pH of around 7.36. Using calcium to buffer the acid is one of the ways in which your body neutralizes it. Therefore, some of the calcium in the dairy products that you ingest is wasted on buffering the acidity of the food and not for other bodily functions, such as building bone density. Many dark green, leafy vegetables, such as broccoli and spinach, are already alkaline, as well as high in calcium, so the calcium ingested from these sources is not wasted on buffering and can be used for improving and maintaining such functions as bone health.

Rule Seven: *Consume Little to No Alcohol*

Every American's favorite pastime seems to include alcohol: sporting events, parties, festivals, a night out with the guys or girls, dinner, and whatever other activity you can think of to include it. Alcohol is a staple in the average person's diet, but does everyone know how much this favorite beverage can sabotage fitness success? Most, I have discovered, do not.

There are seven negative effects alcohol has on your metabolism, especially in relation to added calories:

(1) Remember the phrase I've shared with you throughout this book: *"If you do not use it, you store it."* So when consuming just one drink can equate to anywhere from 140 to over 500 calories, it is not surprising to find out that it is easy to increase your body fat and overall body weight just by having a few drinks a week.

(2) Alcohol also acts like a high glycemic carbohydrate in your system, especially when consuming high sugary drinks, causing huge fluctuations in blood sugar levels that lead to future cravings. If you are talking pure alcohol, it makes most people experience a dip in blood sugar as opposed to a spike.

(3)   It is a nervous system depressant; therefore, it decreases metabolism, and depressing the metabolism is exactly the opposite thing one wants to do when trying to reduce body fat. A high metabolism is critical for successful fat loss so that you are burning any calories you are ingesting.

(4)   Alcohol dehydrates the body, which will slow metabolism even more and dehydrate muscle tissue. Muscle tissue is comprised of about 75 percent water. Therefore, dehydrating this tissue weakens it and can potentially cause muscle loss or the inability to function at optimal levels. This, combined with high glycemic effects and alcohol's diuretic influences on the body, starts the cycle of cravings all over again each time you have a drink. Pure alcohol has no carbs. It does slow fat metabolism, hence the weight gain for heavy drinkers.

(5)   This favorite beverage of the masses reduces protein synthesis, or the building and repair of musculoskeletal tissues. Building and repair of muscle tissue is critical for maintaining and increasing metabolism. The more muscle you have, the leaner and more toned your body will appear; plus, more muscle equates to higher metabolism and increased fat burning capabilities.

(6)   Hormone levels are affected negatively. Exercise increases a variety of hormones in both men and

women, but when consuming alcohol, the secretion of these hormones is reduced dramatically.
Decreases in hormones, such as testosterone
and growth hormones, reduce muscle growth,
repair, and lengthen recovery time.

(7) If those negative effects of alcohol are not
enough to change your mind, then maybe the
hangover will. Being hung over means the quality of your workout is negatively affected. If
the quality of your workouts is affected often
enough, then you will ultimately be burning a
lot less calories in the long run, preventing you
from reaching your personal health and weight-
management goals.

A FEW MORE WORDS ABOUT ALCOHOL

There is something that most people are unaware of
when it comes to alcohol consumption, and that is, just
like proteins, fats, and carbs, alcohol is an energy source
for the body. For each gram of alcohol you consume, it
equates to seven usable calories that your body can use
for normal processes. Knowing this fact, it's important
to keep in mind that regular alcohol consumption can
greatly impact your overall health and personal fitness
goals.

There are two primary views when it comes to consuming alcohol. First is the conventional medical view,
and second is the fitness industry's view. Most people are
aware of the first view but not necessarily the latter of the
two views. Conventional medicine tells us that there are

several health benefits to drinking a glass of red wine a day, which can reduce the risk of heart disease or certain cancers and that it can even raise good cholesterol, or HDL.

Women may consume up to one drink a day, while men can have as many as two. It is also recommended that you do not drink on an empty stomach, so drinking a glass of wine with dinner is good, right? I mean, why not? It is an enjoyable pastime beverage that many Americans enjoy. The problem is that many individuals do not really know about the downside to this popular beverage and why the fitness industry has a completely different view on the topic.

Alcohol, wine especially, is promoted for the wonderful nutrients it provides the body, like phytochemicals that act like antioxidants by preventing free radical damage. Have you ever stopped to think that alcohol comes from natural foods, like grapes, so it is not really the alcohol that is providing those wonderful nutrients but the grapes from which it comes?

What about the cardiovascular disease benefits, like how the resveratrol in wine prevents blood clotting and plaque formation in arteries? But originally resveratrol is found in the skin of grapes, purple grape juice, peanuts, and some berries. Once again, is it the wine that is providing the health benefits, so widely promoted, or the food from which it comes?

What about the harmful effects of alcohol that are not as widely promoted, such as how it increases triglyceride levels and increases the risk of breast cancer in women;

how it can trigger headaches and migraines; its dehydrating effects; how it impairs nutrient absorption, decreases secretion of digestive enzymes from the pancreas, and damages cells lining the stomach and intestines, disabling transport of nutrients into the blood, like water, glucose, sodium, and folate?

What about those next day hangovers? They don't feel so good either. These are just a few of the many harmful side effects alcohol has to offer. If that is not enough to scare you, then how about how it leads to excessive weight gain because of all the empty calories you are consuming with every drink, especially on those nights you don't stop at just drink one or two on top of consuming a full dinner's worth of calories? Plus, you know there's always some late night high calorie heart attack on a plate that always seems to accompany a night out with friends. Grapes and grains do not affect your body this way. They taste good and are good for you; they are what the body needs for optimum health, unlike alcoholic beverages.

Alcohol is toxic to the body. The reason you feel tipsy or get drunk is because it is dehydrating your brain and other bodily cells while inhibiting normal brain activity. You know, the normal brain activity that would usually stop you from putting that lampshade on your head and dancing around like a monkey on espresso. Headaches related to the hangover you feel the next day are a symptom of these damaging effects to the brain.

Because alcohol is a toxin, your body's digestion process is altered as a response to ridding the body of this deadly chemical. For every ounce of alcohol you consume, digestion slows and may even stop for at least one hour or until this substance is eliminated from your blood. Your body will let your food sit in your stomach and intestines longer while it focuses on metabolizing the alcohol in your blood. Alcohol is a poison, and your body knows this, so it tries to get rid of it as quickly as possible in an effort to protect itself and the health and vitality of its cells.

One of the reasons alcoholics have distended stomachs is not only due to liver swelling but because their intestines are full of feces that cannot be eliminated properly. This may not necessarily mean they are constipated in the normal sense; they usually eliminate pretty regularly. The problem is that there is food that gets stuck in their body, which is just rotting in their intestines. This is old stuff due to improper elimination related to drinking regularly. To a lesser degree, this happens to you each time you decide to drink on a full stomach.

Sound appealing yet?

What about the excessive calories that lead to weight gain? In the next chapter, you will learn that your body only needs a few hundred calories every few hours for proper weight management. If you are reading this book, then you most likely realize that serving size is something you should take into consideration when addressing weight loss goals.

Keeping this in mind, let us say that you ate a well-balanced meal that encompassed the proper servings, serving sizes, and caloric needs for attaining your weight loss goals. What about the alcohol you are drinking with your dinner or shortly after? Did you take that into consideration? Each drink you consume can equate to anywhere from 120 calories, such as a glass of wine, to 500 or more from those fancy mixed drinks. What this means is that once you use the calories you need from the initial alcohol calories consumed, the rest of those alcohol calories, plus all of your meal calories, will now be stored as fat. Your body only needs a few hundred calories every three hours, and you may have just consumed enough calories for the entire day from dinner and a couple of drinks. Are you starting to get the picture of where those extra fat pounds came from now?

Fitness competitors and many avid fitness professionals will tell you to reduce and even eliminate alcohol from your diet entirely for the best physical and energetic benefits. Alcohol prevents muscle growth along with proper healing, and it leads to increased fat pounds. As a former fitness competitor, I know that it is completely impossible to have a strong influence on fat reduction if I consume alcohol when trying to get lean. In preparation for a competition, alcohol is at the top of the list for things to go. The other aspect of differences in opinion lies with the recommendation that you should eat a meal before drinking.

The conventional approach to alcohol encourages food because it slows the rate at which alcohol is absorbed into the bloodstream. The downside to this is that people usually drink more as a result. In the fitness industry, it is common for competitors to drink alcohol without eating a meal first, on the rare occasions they choose to drink. This eliminates a ton of excess calories.

If you decide to take the fitness industry approach to alcohol, be aware that if you drink on an empty stomach, you'll feel the effects of the alcohol more quickly, and it will be stronger than usual. Therefore, be cautious to drink slowly and less than you normally do. In fact, you should not drink more than one to two drinks maximum because it could lead to stomach irritation and unexpected drunkenness due to the alcohol's faster absorption rate when food is not present in the stomach.

If you decide to take this approach, be sure to eat food at least two to three hours prior to drinking, and wait about three hours after you finished drinking to allow your body to thoroughly digest the alcohol you already consumed. This will give your body the necessary time needed to metabolize your food and alcohol without causing an overlap of calories and slowed digestion. Plus, by the time you're ready to eat again, after you're finished having a drink or two, your buzz will have worn off.

This way, you will make better food choices, instead of the normal high calorie ones that usually accompany a few drinks. In the end, if you try this approach, you'll consume a lot less calories during a night out, which will allow you to have fun and yet still reach your goals.

These two opposing views are just that. It does not mean that one group is right and the other is wrong; it just means that they have different outcome-driven approaches to the same topic.

What about me? Well, I decided around age twenty-five to completely eliminate alcohol from my diet, just to see what the results were and because I was serious about competing and knew I wouldn't be able to if I didn't. I was truly amazed by how much healthier I felt and how much better my body looked after eliminating alcohol completely. I can't explain how challenging it was to make this choice because it seems like our entire society and all social events seem to revolve around the consumption of alcohol.

Weekends for me used to always be hanging out with friends at various events and drinking. Not excessively, but at least a few nights a week. Sometimes I'd even come home from a hard day's work and have a glass of wine to relax. For about six months, I chose not to even go in bars to help me achieve my goal of no alcohol. My friends gave me such a hard time, but I stuck with it, and I'm really glad I did. I completely eliminated it for about two years, and wow, did I feel good, and my physique evolved to a whole new level of fit.

I was so healthy during that time that I didn't even catch a cold. I do drink on occasion now, but I can tell you that it is only max about one time a month. But a lot of times months will go by without me having a drink, and I can say that I don't really miss it. I feel so good when it's not in my diet that it's an easy change to live with. When it comes to alcohol consumption, you need to make the best decision for you and your lifestyle, so hopefully this will give you some insight so that you can do that in a way that aids you in attaining your goals.

Rule Eight: *Consume Two to Four Servings of Protein throughout the Day*

The only source of protein your body has available for use during the day, other than what you receive from your diet, is that which makes up muscle fibers and other soft tissues of the body. Therefore, it is imperative for you to consume protein periodically throughout the day in an effort to maintain a positive nitrogen balance so that your body does not break down muscle tissue for needed protein and nitrogen to use in the healing processes of the body.

Eating protein frequently throughout the day also has another benefit, and that is to keep appetite at bay. Due to the fact that carbohydrates cause fluctuation in blood sugar levels, they will cause you to feel hungrier more often. When consuming protein, due to their lack of effect on blood sugar levels and the length of time it takes to break them down to useable nutrients, they cause you to feel more satisfied longer throughout the day. This benefit prevents overeating and keeps energy levels at a higher and more consistent level throughout the day.

Rule Nine: *Rotate Your Calories*

Your body and its metabolism adjust to any regular dietary patterns you practice consistently. Initial weight loss from calorie-restricted diets occurs due to your calorie consumption being less than your current metabolic rate. However, the fast and extreme weight loss results that you normally experience at the beginning of this type of diet have a tendency to diminish within a short period.

The reason for this is that your body adjusts your metabolism by breaking down muscle, which, in turn, slows the metabolic rate of the body permanently *unless* you rebuild the lost muscle tissue sometime in the future. When you consume a set number of calories each day, your metabolism gets used to this number and adjusts your metabolic rate accordingly. Your body is always trying to find a balance because maintaining extreme calorie restriction over an extended period could lead to too much weight loss and therefore death, so the body makes these alterations to prevent health problems in the future. This is why extreme changes should be avoided. Subtle changes over time will keep your body from becoming alarmed and adjusting your metabolism.

A prime example of extreme states of change that is not necessarily healthy for your body is when consuming a high protein, low carbohydrate diet. These types of diets, where one vital nutrient needed for life maintenance is drastically reduced to unhealthy norms, will cause your body to become very efficient at utilizing the little carbs you are receiving.

When you start eating carbs again, a major rebound effect occurs because your body is so efficient at utilizing the carbs that were once minimal in your diet. What happens here is that after your diet returns to normal, you blow up like a balloon with symptoms, such as water retention and quick fat storage, because of your body's efficiency to use the little carbs you were getting.

When you throw your body back out of whack via a drastic restriction such as this, it will cause physiological and other imbalances that take days or even weeks for it to adjust to those changes and find balance once again. Balance, in this case, would be to receive the correct balance of fats, proteins, and carbohydrates. When your body returns to a normal carb, fat, and protein ratio after a restriction such as this, again it may take up to a few weeks for your body to adjust and for water balance, carb utilization, and other alterations to return to normal.

Adjustments to your diet should be subtle, and when it comes to calorie consumption, calories need to be inconsistent so as to keep your body guessing. The key is to prevent your metabolism from adjusting to fewer calories in your diet, and the best way to accomplish this is by rotating them.

To do this, you will want to consume anywhere from one hundred to three hundred fewer calories in a day, 60 to 75 percent of the time, making sure to rotate the number of calories. Then, on some weeks, you can reduce them by five hundred calories at least one day on some weeks and two days on others.

Have a cheat day anywhere from one to four days a month, which will help to boost your metabolism and keep it running higher in an effort to prevent it from decreasing for those days where calories are lower. Increasing the number of calories you burn on a consistent basis will also help to keep your metabolism running higher.

Fitness Rules Reflected

I know that you may be thinking at this point, *Wow, is that strict!* The thing to keep in mind and the reason I've told you about these fitness industry rules that competitors follow is so that you can be aware of what it takes to get in competitor shape. It doesn't mean you have to do all of them or even some of them, but you can take them into consideration and maybe meet at a point somewhere in between that is right for you.

If you're someone who is just looking for a few tips to get you past a plateau, then use these as guidelines to make subtle adjustments to your current nutritional plan. If you're someone who is looking to take it to the next level, a level that may be beyond the average person's physique, then you may want to implement all of these rules to the fullest into your personal plan.

For all of you, I just wanted you to learn some concepts that you may not have been aware of, which could aid you in attaining your goals faster and with more ease than that of past efforts. Take these tips and approach them in a way that's best for you and your current fitness goals and lifestyle.

READING FOOD LABELS

Reading labels can save your life.

Think about it: you have probably read the labels on just about everything, from household appliances to chemicals you use to clean your car. You do this for a number of reasons. Sometimes you read labels to know why or how something works or what is in it. You may read labels to prevent injury while using certain products. You wouldn't pick up a bottle of Drano and drink it before you read the label ensuring it is safe to drink, would you? Of course not.

The real question here is, do you ever really take the time to read about the foods you eat every day? If you have, do you understand what it is you are reading? Unfortunately, many people do not. You might be thinking that ingesting food is not going to poison you like drinking Drano would, but don't be so sure. Some of the additives in our foods can be toxic, especially when consumed in large doses.

In most cases, people do not really think about what they eat prior to consuming it. People choose the foods they eat for a variety of reasons, such as taste, boredom, cravings, limited choices, convenience, social pressures, emotional cues, or physiological needs, like dehydration or low blood sugar levels.

So why is it important to read labels before you take that first scrumptious bite? Well, what if I told you that you could be consuming poison? That's right, poison. The food and liquids you have ingested over the years have created the body you live in today, and either that body is healthy or it is sick.

A healthy body can move freely; it feels good, possesses an abundance of vitality and stamina, sleeps well, and feels refreshed upon awakening. There are no health problems, no need for medications, and your physique is not overweight or obese. On the other hand, an unhealthy body, well, you get the picture. You really *are* what you eat! Understanding which foods create health and which foods create sickness and disease starts with reading and understanding food labels.

In a perfect world, every meal every day would consist of one-ingredient fresh foods. In this world, you would also sleep eight hours a night, vacation six to twelve weeks a year, work no more than four hours a day at a job you absolutely love, and eat six small meals a day using foods picked from your own garden and prepared fresh in your own kitchen.

This is actually the way life is meant to be, enjoyable and healthy. For the most part, we do want to eat an abundance of one-ingredient fresh foods, but realistically, it may not always be possible. The key is that when you do have to eat from a box, a can, a jar, a tube, or even a drive-thru bag, it is important to understand what it is that you are really eating. Comprehending food labels and knowing what to look for is critical for making proactive dietary choices.

Disease or Poisoning?

There are a number of diseases found to be increasing year after year, which include:

- Fibromyalgia
- Epilepsy
- Lupus
- Arthritis
- Alzheimer's disease
- Lymphoma

- Multiple Sclerosis (MS)
- Birth defects
- Attention Deficit Disorder (ADD and ADHD)
- Overweight and obesity
- Panic disorder
- Parkinson's disease
- Lyme disease
- Chronic Fatigue Syndrome
- Multiple Chemical Sensitivities (MCS)
- Depression and other psychological disorders
- Diabetes and diabetic complications

I ask you, are these diseases or toxicity from the everyday foods you eat? You may ask, what does this have to do with weight loss or reading labels? I say everything. These days, being overweight or obese is classified as a disease. In truth, it is an imbalance of the body rather than a disease that you have no control over. Therefore, being overweight is not the problem but only a symptom of an unbalanced lifestyle and poor nutritional habits. Being overweight is the effect of being biochemically, emotionally, physically, and spiritually out of a healthy equilibrium.

Eating foods with additives that increase the shelf life or enhance the flavor of that food and that the body does not need causes biochemical imbalances, resulting in dis-ease (a body out of whack) or disease (a sickness). Knowing which additives can cause health-related problems can be tricky. A good rule of thumb is if you're reading the ingredients list and you can't pronounce some of the ingredients or you don't know what they are, then don't eat the item. Know what you are sticking in your mouth because it could be inhibiting you from weight loss success or worse, like damaging your health.

Bring the body's chemistry back to balance with a healthy eating plan, and you will eliminate the symptoms associated with the dis-ease, disease, or pain associated with the imbalance. In doing this, you will ultimately eliminate the symptoms associated with the body's unhealthy physiology, such as disease, anxiety, depression, musculoskeletal pain, fatigue, lack of vitality, low stamina, weight gain, overweight, and obesity.

How Much is Too Much?

Not only is eating the right kind of food important for weight loss, but eating the right amounts of your food choices are just as important as well. If you are anything like my son, for instance, you may get one of the biggest bowls available in the house and fill it to the top with cereal in the morning or for a late night snack. This usually equates to half a family size box and well over what a recommended serving is.

For a growing boy, this may be okay, but for someone interested in creating a lean physique, it is definitely not. When your goals are focused on weight loss, it is important to look at the serving sizes of the food you eat. When it comes to the foods you eat every day, do you even know what a serving consists of? Are you eating enough or too much at one sitting?

The average male needs approximately 2000 calories a day, while the average female needs 1500 calories daily. Divide that by three meals and three snacks a day, and you get three hundred to four hundred calories at main meals for men and two hundred to three hundred calories at main meals for women. As for snacks, men might consume two hundred to three hundred calorie snacks and women one hundred to two hundred ones. Metabolism is unique to each individual, so you may eat more or less calories to suit your lifestyle, activity, and unique health and fitness goals.

As mentioned earlier, it is important to eat every three hours for maintaining a high metabolism, but keep in mind that your meals and snacks should equate to just enough to meet your lifestyle and energy needs. Remember, walking away from a meal feeling full means that you are storing fat.

To give your body just enough (no more, no less), you will need to stick to single serving sizes, therefore eating only until you have a feeling of contentment. Thinking back, how many times have you walked away from a meal feeling full? I bet it is more times than you can count. This may be just one reason of many as to why you may be struggling with your weight today.

Start reading the labels of the foods you eat on a daily basis and find out whether you are eating enough or too much per sitting. The best way to determine this is by measuring the amount of food you eat for at least a week, or until you get in the habit of eating only one serving per sitting or enough to suit your calorie needs.

Let us take a look at a basic food label and review some tips for making good choices. The nutrition facts on the food label to the left provide you with information about certain nutrients available in the product so that you can make proactive dietary decisions. Your body needs the right combination of nutrients for optimal health. The nutrition facts food panel is printed somewhere on the outside of every packaged food, easily accessible for the consumer's view.

Nutrition Facts

Serving Size 8 crackers (31g)
(1 serving = 2 full cracker sheets)
Servings Per Container About 13

Amount Per Serving

Calories 120   Calories from Fat 15

	% Daily Value*
Total Fat 2g	3%
Saturated Fat 0g	0%
Trans Fat 0g	
Polyunsaturated Fat 1g	
Monounsaturated Fat 0g	
Cholesterol 0mg	0%
Sodium 190mg	8%
Potassium 45mg	1%
Total Carbohydrate 25g	8%
Dietary Fiber 1g	4%
Sugars 8g	
Protein 2g	

Vitamin A 0%	•	Vitamin C 0%
Calcium 15%	•	Iron 6%

*Percent Daily Values are based on a 2,000 calorie diet. Your daily values may be higher or lower depending on your calorie needs:

	Calories:	2,000	2,500
Total Fat	Less than	65g	80g
Sat Fat	Less than	20g	25g
Cholesterol	Less than	300mg	300mg
Sodium	Less than	2,400mg	2,400mg
Potassium		3,500mg	3,500mg
Total Carbohydrate		300g	375g
Dietary Fiber		25g	30g

The nutrients on food labels are measured in grams (g) and milligrams (mg). There are one thousand milligrams in a gram. Other information on the label is given in percentages. These numbers are based on eating two thousand calories in a day.

A calorie is a unit of energy, a way of expressing how much energy your body absorbs by ingesting this product or how much energy it will take to burn off the food you just ate. To learn more about reading food labels, take a look below. The descriptions will refer to the information on the label from the top in a descending order to bottom.

SERVING SIZES

The nutrition label always lists the amount of a serving size, such as one cup of cereal or one slice of bread. You will also find what percentage or amount of nutrients is in one serving.

SERVING PER CONTAINER OR PACKAGE

Servings per container are the number of servings in the entire package, based on the described serving size portion. If there are ten servings in a box of cookies and each serving is one cookie, then there will be a total of ten cookies in the entire box.

CALORIES AND CALORIES FROM FAT

The number of calories in a single serving is listed on the left side of the label. You will also find the total number of calories that come from fat directly next to the total calories. Choosing naturally low-fat choices will aid in weight loss because less fat means less calories to burn later.

PERCENT DAILY VALUE

The percent daily values, located on the right side of the label, refer to the recommended percentage of daily allowances, based on a two thousand-calorie diet. This means the amount recommended by the USDA for optimum health.

For instance, there is a recommended daily allowance for fat, so the food label might say that one serving of this food meets 10 percent of your daily fat needs, based on a two thousand-calorie adult diet. What your needs are (based on a two thousand-calorie diet) is listed at the bottom of every label. Percentages of daily values include total carbohydrate, fiber, total fat, saturated fat, cholesterol, sodium, vitamin A, vitamin C, iron, and calcium.

TOTAL FAT

The total fat is the number of fat grams contained in one serving. The different types of fat are saturated, unsaturated (monounsaturated and polyunsaturated), and trans fat, and each are listed separately on the label.

CHOLESTEROL AND SODIUM

These numbers tell you how much cholesterol and sodium (salt) are in a single serving.

TOTAL CARBOHYDRATE

This number tells you how many carbohydrates are in one serving. Carbohydrates are broken down into grams of fiber and sugar as well.

PROTEIN

This number tells you how much protein is in each serving.

VITAMINS A AND C

This list shows the percent daily value of vitamin A and C available in each serving.

CALCIUM AND IRON

This list shows the percent daily value of calcium and iron in a serving.

ADDED SUGARS

There are varieties of sweeteners that manufacturers add to foods that may or may not have an effect on your weight loss results. Look for these added sugars and sweeteners in the ingredients section. The ingredients are listed in order from the most abundant to the least abundant ingredient in the product (it actually goes by weight). Here is a list of sweeteners to look for:

- Brown sugar
- Corn sweetener
- Dextrose

- Fructose
- Glucose
- Maltose
- Lactose
- High-fructose corn syrup
- Corn syrup
- Corn syrup solids
- Malt syrup
- Raw sugar
- Sugar
- Stevia
- Molasses
- Aspartame
- NutraSweet
- Equal
- Sunette
- Splenda
- Sucrose
- Sucralose
- Saccharin
- Mannitol
- Sorbitol
- Xylitol
- Lactitol
- Isomalt
- Maltitol
- Hydrogenated starch hydrolysates (HSH)

FOOD LABEL TIPS

When reading food labels, it is important to look to the most abundant macronutrient between fat, protein, and carbs. Many people believe that nuts and nut butter are a great source of protein, but in actuality, they are more of a fat source than a protein source—albeit a *good* fat source.

You will find this by checking the number of grams of each nutrient in each serving. As an example, one serving of your average peanut butter has seventeen grams of fat, seven grams of carbohydrate, and seven grams of protein. As you can see, the most prevalent macronutrient between the three is fat. Therefore, peanut butter is a great source of good or unsaturated fats but not the best source of protein. Keeping this in mind, choose foods according to their highest nutrient base for the meal plan tracking checklist.

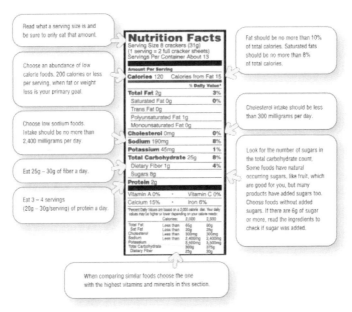

OTHER SIMPLE TIPS
TO KEEP IN MIND

- When using eggs in your meal preparations, you can substitute two egg whites for one whole egg. The yolks consist mostly of fat, which will add extra undesirable calories to your diet.

- For scrambled eggs or omelets, you may want to use mostly egg whites with only one to two egg yolks to create lower calorie meals.

- Many dairy products, such as yogurt or ice cream, have added sugars (dairy also has natural sugars in the form of lactose). They may be in the form of high-fructose corn syrup, dextrose, and/or other sugars. This is true for most processed and prepared supermarket foods. Extra sugar in food accounts for a large amount of excess calories and no nutritional value. Be sure to read food labels for added ingredients. If you choose to keep dairy in your diet, there are a wide variety of "No Sugar Added" dairy products now available to help you make better nutritional choices.

- If you have a hard time getting enough protein in your diet, remember, you can use protein supplements (natural varieties are best). Choose one sweetened with Stevia or low in sugars (five grams or less per serving). Try a few different varieties; some taste better than others do. But remember that getting your protein from whole foods is best.

- When shopping for fruit juices, look for 100 percent juice with no added sugar.

- Did you know it is better to eat a piece of fruit than it is to drink a glass of fruit juice? It takes at least four to six oranges to make one glass of juice. That is a lot of calories, plus you miss out on all that natural fiber.

- Sweet potatoes and yams are higher in fiber and other nutrients than white potatoes.

- When buying vegetables, choose a wide variety of colors. Certain vegetables are higher in selected vitamins than others, so choosing an array of colors will ensure a good balance of vitamin intake.

- Be creative with your meals. Using salsa, light soy sauce, lemon or other fruit juices, and/or spices, you can add a lot of flavor without excess fat or calories. Using fruit is also another great way to spice up a meal. One recipe example of this is Hawaiian chicken, grilled chicken with teriyaki sauce and sliced pineapple.

- The key to permanent weight loss is working to develop healthier eating habits. If you bring home foods high in calories, fat, and sugar that add little nutritional value to your diet, then you will only slow progress and end up discouraged.

MEAL PLANNING

Taking into consideration all of the information from step four, it is now time to create some healthy meal plans to help you stay on track toward reaching your personal fitness goals. Here is a simple guideline to follow when planning future meals:

- Choose mostly one-ingredient fresh foods.
- Remember, when it comes to vegetables, fresh is best, frozen next, and try to refrain from canned foods.
- Choose naturally low-fat foods.
- Consume fruits before 2:00 p.m. so that you can utilize calories for activities and rehydrate your system.
- Consume complex carbohydrates, including whole grains, multigrain cereals, and beans by 4:00 p.m. so that you burn these high-energy foods off before the end of the day instead of storing them.
- Consume proteins and veggies all day long:
  - Vegetables throughout the day will keep you feeling satisfied all day long; they also prevent overeating and give you an abundance of natural energy due to the vitamins and minerals and other nutrients these foods provide the body.
  - Periodically consuming protein throughout the day will help you to feel satisfied throughout the day, along with maintaining positive nitrogen balance for soft tis-

sue, muscle, and other cellular repair and healing.

- Drink one gallon of water a day.
- Consume little to no added sugars.
- Try to shoot for these servings of various foods throughout each day for best fat-loss results (see servings sizes below):
  ° Four to six vegetables
  ° Two to four proteins
  ° One to two fruits
  ° Two to three whole grains
  ° Minimal added fats
- Use the meal planning tables on the following pages to help you make good nutritional decisions based on the information presented in this section. If you're eating the wrong types of foods during certain times of the day, try the first table to ensure you are making more appropriate time-based selections. If consuming too many calories seems to be more of a problem for you, then try tracking calories, along with fat, protein, and carbohydrate grams.

Meal Plan Checklist

Source	Servings	Food Groups and Serving Sizes

Source (vertical labels): Fruits Until 2 PM · Whole Grains & Fats Until 4 PM · Proteins & Vegetables All Day Long

Meal #1　Time:
- ☐ Whole Grain
- ☐ Fruit or Protein
- ☐ Water
- ☐ Water

Snack　Time:
- ☐ Fruit or Protein
- ☐ Healthy Fat
- ☐ Water
- ☐ Water

Meal #2　Time:
- ☐ Vegetables
- ☐ Whole Grain
- ☐ Protein
- ☐ Water

Snack　Time:
- ☐ Protein and/or Vegetables
- ☐ Water

Meal #3　Time:
- ☐ Vegetables
- ☐ Protein
- ☐ Water

Snack　Time:
- ☐ Vegetables and/or Protein
- ☐ Water

Food Groups and Serving Sizes

PROTEIN (2 – 4 Servings Daily)

20 – 30 grams = Serving Size

Meat, Fish, Eggs, Poultry
3 – 4 oz = Serving Size
Size of the palm of your hand in diameter
and I inch thick

Protein Drinks
1 – 1½ Scoops
20 – 30 Grams

Best Protein Sources – **Grade A**
Poultry, Fish, Lean Beef, Egg Whites

Mediocre Protein Sources – **Grade B**
Protein Supplements (Must be high protein and
very low carbs to be considered protein drinks),
Soy Products (Unsweetened soy milk & tofu)

Low Quality Protein Sources – **Grade C**
Dairy Products, Nuts, Other Soy Products
Protein Supplements (Bars & drinks high in carbs)

WHOLE GRAINS (2 – 3 Servings Daily)

½ – ¾ cup = Serving Size
Brown Rice, Oatmeal, High Fiber Cereals,
Yams, Legumes (Beans), Lentils, Quinoa

HEALTHY FATS (1 – 2 Servings Daily)
Not to Reflect Total Daily Fat Grams

5g = Serving Size
Avocados, Unsalted Raw Nuts & Seeds,
Green & Black Olives, Healthy Unsaturated Oils

VEGETABLES (4 – 6 Servings Daily)

¾ – 1 cup – Serving Size

FRUITS (1 – 2 Servings Daily)

1 Small Medium Piece
Or
½ – 1 cup = Serving Size

WATER (8 – 10 Servings Daily)

8 oz = Serving Size

Meal Plan Tracking

Source	Food & Preparation	Calories	Fat	Protein	Sugar	Fiber
Fruits Until 2 PM / Whole Grains & Fats Until 4 PM / Proteins & Vegetables All Day Long	**Meal #1** Time:					
	Snack Time:					
	Meal #2 Time:					
	Snack Time: 3 PM					
	Meal #3 Time: 6 PM					
	Snack Time: 9 PM					

GROCERY SHOPPING

The most important goal when grocery shopping is to buy mainly one-ingredient natural and alive foods. When purchasing prepackaged foods, a tip to keep in mind is that if you cannot pronounce the ingredients listed on the box or if you do not know what those ingredients are, do not eat it! Buy natural, one-ingredient foods like apples, oranges, chicken breasts, steaks, oatmeal, et cetera. It is what your body was designed to digest, not something out of a box with fifty foreign ingredients you cannot even pronounce.

When you do your grocery shopping, only buy healthy food! Leave the junk food at the store. The more junk food you eat, the more you will want, so do not bring any home. Focus on new, healthy foods. Be creative by using natural ingredients to sweeten your foods and herbs to put some kick into your meals. Who said eating healthy had to be dull anyway?

This doesn't mean you can never cheat; it just means that you should not cheat every day. Try making a cheat day a special event that you enjoy with your friends or family. Go out to a special place and just eat dessert for dinner one night, or invite a group of friends over for ice cream and brownie creations, and make sure all the junk food is gone before they leave. This makes it harder for you to cheat and sabotage the positive progress you have made while creating the opportunity to bond with friends and family. This is definitely a win-win to me, and I've done this many times in the past with my own friends and family. It's also a great way to keep junk out of the house without everyone getting upset about it.

SUMMING IT UP

Step four focuses on implementing what you have learned in both steps three and four. The Understanding Nutrition and Meal Planning sections have given you the information you need so that you may be able to plan and prepare more proactive menus geared toward attaining your personal fat-loss and fitness goals.

Initially, changes to your eating habits will need to be a conscientious process and require time commitment for planning. However, with time and practice over the next few weeks, this process of change will become easier and evolve into positive lifestyle habits.

You will also begin experiencing the results of your efforts, reinforcing these new dietary habits. The next step reviews information on proper exercise and its importance in the weight loss formula, so read on and find out why exercise is a critical component to getting fit.

STEP 5:

Exercise 101

No way of thinking about your health could ever be complete without including exercise in the planning process. While the "mind versus muscle" debate has raged for centuries, in my mind there is no debate: you simply can't have one without the other. For your mind to function properly, your body must function properly. Conversely, if you want to be at your best physically, you must also be at your best mentally.

Accordingly, step five focuses on the basic components of exercise that encompass a well-balanced program. Like nutrition, exercise also has a number of elements that are necessary for attaining a fit body.

These four components include:

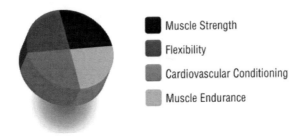

Muscle Strength

Flexibility

Cardiovascular Conditioning

Muscle Endurance

Failure to include all four of these branches into your program may result in muscle imbalances and poor overall health of the heart, lungs, body, bones, tendons, and ligaments.

In step five, you will also learn about exercise intensity and how to determine what intensity is best for you based upon your individual fitness level, fitness goals, and personal needs.

After you finish reading this section, the various components of exercise and their importance will no longer be a mystery to you. You will feel comfortable knowing you are doing it the right way, and your results will speak for themselves.

THINKING FIT EQUALS BEING FIT

Before we dig deeper into this chapter, I want to remind you that health is a way of life. Unfortunately, many people feel they can be healthy without being fit. But ask yourself, does that really make sense?

While you *do* have to *Think Fit 2 Be Fit*, you can't literally "think yourself fit." So this chapter is where the mind meets the muscle, and frankly, it's not always pleasant. Exercise can be challenging, even demanding, but it is also rewarding in so many ways, and as a mature, intelligent adult, I know you know what I'm talking about.

So often we're too smart for our own good. By that I mean rather than just simply getting up and doing something (because we know it's good for our bodies and we'll feel better about it later), we let the negative chatter in our heads talk us out of it. We have to make a conscious effort to eliminate the negative mental chatter and replace it with positive self-talk that encourages us to move, even when we don't think we want to. This is truly when you can *Think Fit 2 Be Fit* because you literally out-think the negative self-talk and replace it with positive words *and* actions to add the healthy benefit of exercise to your daily routine.

The key with exercise is that once you actually start moving, your body will release hormones, like endorphins, that create changes in the way you feel—both mentally and physically. The hormones released in your system due to exercise not only elevate your mood but have a pain blocking effect, so not only will you feel happier, your body will feel better in a multitude of ways too.

Have you ever noticed that when you first start jogging (or lifting weights or bicycling or playing tennis or whatever), you're a little stiff, a little negative, a little disbelieving that you can actually complete the mile or the course or the game, set, and match? And then, after only a few minutes, your mind-set changes to feel more positive, your muscles and joints limber up, and you actually start to feel good? Well, thank your hormones! On top of all those healthy benefits, your positive attitude will be exacerbated because you'll know the outcome will be well worth it.

TARGET HEART RATE (THR)

No one can tell you exactly how hard to work out, how long to work out, or, for that matter, what to do as part of your workout. Exercise is individual to each, well ... individual! Who you are, your body type, your age, your job, your family status, your schedule, even your sex will determine what type, intensity, and duration of exercise you should engage in.

And, since fitness levels differ from individual to individual, it is important to monitor and adjust your exercise intensity by monitoring and using your heart rate as a guide. Monitoring your heart rate and adjusting the intensity of your workout accordingly will ensure you are working at the correct intensity for your fitness level and goals.

Target heart rate (THR) is one of the most important fitness tools you can use to make sure you are personalizing your specific exercise routine for your specific needs. It is the number one aid for determining if you are working too hard or too light. For instance, have you ever noticed those individuals at the gym that exercise every day yet years later they are still overweight and look as if they have made no progress at all? In many cases, this is because they are just not working out at the right intensity, and unfortunately, they are completely unaware of why they never make any progress.

The number one reason why people do not make progress is due to working at the wrong exercise intensity, which can only be determined by monitoring heart rate. I have seen several individuals in gyms over the years that are just not training in the right heart rate zone to produce the results they want. The key to success is working out in a way that gets you *the results you want.*

The *only* way to determine if you are doing something right is via monitoring, analyzing, and then adjusting your program in accordance with the data you receive. You need a point, or several points, of reference to accomplish this task.

The most prominent and accurate means of determining target heart rate is by the **Karvonen formula**. This formula calculates a percentage of the heart rate reserve, which is the difference between the resting heart rate and the maximal heart rate. Heart rate reserve equals the maximal heart rate minus resting heart rate. Let's examine this formula a little more closely:

- **Maximal heart rate** is the highest rate a person can attain during exercise.
- Maximal heart rate equals 220 minus your age.

This formula is based on the assumption that one's heart rate at birth is 220 and decreases one beat per minute every year. **Resting heart rate** is the rate at which your heart beats at full rest. It is recommended that this rate be taken before getting out of bed in the morning (while you are as close to "rest" as possible).

To find your resting heart rate, find your pulse then count the number of heartbeats you feel for a full sixty seconds. Repeat this for three consecutive mornings and then find your average by adding your results for each day and dividing that number by three to find your average resting heart rate (RHR).

To determine exercise intensity, use the **Karvonen formula:**

- 220 - age = maximal heart rate
- MHR - RHR = heart rate reserve (HRR)
- HRR x intensity level + RHR = target heart rate (THR)

The generally accepted heart rate ranges are between 60 and 70 percent for the fat burning zone or between 70 and 80 percent for the cardiovascular zone. Take a look at how you would calculate target heart rate for someone forty-five years old that has a resting heart rate of eighty beats per minute. The target heart rate is 80 percent of maximal HRR.

HR Key:

HR = Heart Rate

THR = Target Heart Rate

RHR = Resting Heart Rate

HRR = Heart Rate Reserve

MHR = Max Heart Rate

THR = [(MHR - RHR) x % Intensity] + RHR

EXAMPLE:

220 - 45 = 175	220 - Age = MHR
175 - 75 = 100	MHR - RHR = HRR
100 x .80 + 75 = 155	(HRR x % Intensity) + RHR = THR

Warm-Up

HRR x 40% = _____ + Resting HR = _____ This is your max Target HR

HRR x 60% = _____ + Resting HR= _____ This is your min Target HR

Fat Burning Zone

HRR x 60% = _____ + Resting HR= _____ This is your min Target HR

HRR x 70% = _____ + Resting HR= _____ This is your max Target HR

Cardio Zone

HRR x 70% = _____ + Resting HR= _____ This is your min Target HR

HRR x 80% = _____ + Resting HR= _____ This is your max Target HR

The **Karvonen formula** is considered to be a more accurate formula for determining exercise intensity than the **maximal heart rate formula**, which is 220 - age x intensity. The MHR formula does not take into consideration a person's current fitness level via using their resting heart rate when formulating heart rate zones, whereas the Karvonen formula does.

WORKOUT DYNAMICS

When we say "workout," what do we mean? Well, everybody has a different opinion. For some, gardening in the morning is a workout, while for others training for an upcoming triathalon is a workout. The fact is both are right, *if* what they consider a workout contains the building blocks of what I call "workout dynamics."

What are workout dynamics? The actual dynamics of every workout are basically the same. What this means is that regardless of the type of training you have chosen to reach your fitness goals, each workout follows the format of first warming up, ROM exercise or stretching, core workout, and cooling down.

Start any activity at approximately 50 percent your peak core workout intensity and progress by gradually increasing the intensity, resistance, and/or workload over the course of the workout, practice session, or activity of choice. Follow this cycle: lower intensity warm-up, ROM exercise or light stretching, core work, and cool down.

Warming Up

One of the best ways to think about fitness is to see it as a lifelong habit, as much a part of your life as brushing your teeth or taking a shower. Most of us talk about "getting fit" or "getting pumped" or "getting toned," but we have to shift our mind-set (*Think Fit 2 Be Fit*) to see fitness as a *state of being*. In other words, we shouldn't get fit; we should be fit. We shouldn't get toned; we should be toned.

Our national "get fit" mentality causes a lot of my students to end up in ankle braces and casts because they go from zero to sixty in a single day. They play the *Rocky* theme, run too far, too fast, too long, and collapse with shin splints, cramps, dehydration, heat exhaustion—or give up because it's too hard. All because of their desire to "get" somewhere they should already "be."

Warming up is a way of easing ourselves into the habit of flexibility, which, of course, leads to the other three habits we need to acquire to truly be fit: muscular endurance, muscular strength, and cardiovascular fitness. Warming up is an important part of any exercise program because it prepares the body for exercise. Preparing the body for exercise makes exercise more comfortable and decreases the possible risk of injuries. The purpose of warming up is to increase all of the following:

- Blood pressure
- Oxygen consumption
- Dilation of blood vessels
- Flexibility of the working muscles

- Body temperature
- Overall circulation

Increased circulation allows blood and nutrients to flow to the working muscles, giving them the energy they need to perform work. Your warm-up should consist of five to fifteen minutes of low intensity aerobic activity, which may include walking, jogging, stair climbing, cycling, marching in place, or any other low intensity activity that increases your heart rate.

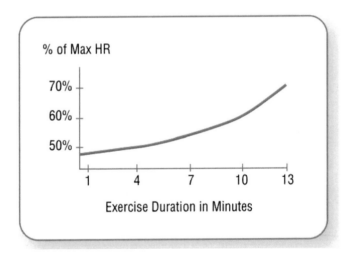

When warming up, begin at a low intensity, around 40 to 50 percent of your MHR, and gradually increase intensity toward the end of the warm-up until you reach approximately 60 to 70 percent of your MHR. This aids in the prevention of too much lactic acid being released in your body and working muscles during your workout.

Lactic acid is a byproduct of exercise, causing onset of localized muscle fatigue, which can limit the duration and intensity of your overall workout. Although you may not recognize its name, this pesky byproduct is a major culprit in causing muscle burn, pre-fatigue, and delayed onset of soreness. Therefore, warming up correctly will reduce and may even eliminate delayed soreness following exercise.

Some other benefits of a good warm-up include:

- Increases kinesthetic awareness (hand-eye-coordination), a protection mechanism that helps to reduce the risk of potential injuries
- Psychological preparation (mental readiness)
- Increased enthusiasm

Stretching or Range of Motion (ROM) Exercises

What if you could avoid the aches, pains, and strains of overexerting yourself, or worse, not preparing yourself for exercise in the first place? You can, you know, with something I'll be teaching you in this section called range of motion (or ROM) exercises.

Many people think that the sequence to an exercise routine starts with stretching. This could not be further from the truth. Warming up is the first step in your *preparation to exercise*. ROM exercises, or stretching, come directly *after* your warm-up, once your body temperature has risen and circulation has increased, therefore making muscles more flexible and less likely to be injured.

After a warm-up is the perfect time to lightly stretch the muscles and prepare the joints for the activity you will be participating in. Light stretching helps prepare the ligaments, tendons, and muscles for the work that lies ahead. Stretching after a warm-up is usually much lighter than the stretching that you perform post-workout for cool down and flexibility reasons. Light stretching is recommended before cardiovascular workouts and light ROM exercise before weight training.

Range of motion exercise, or ROM, is exercise that is done with little to no weight in preparation to lift heavier weights. For instance, if you were training chest, prior to lifting the normal heavier sets in your routine, you would start by performing one to two sets of the same exercise but at 50 percent of your max weight. You will be performing the same exact exercise but at a much lighter weight, taking your body through a normal chest ROM. The benefit of doing so will allow you to lightly stretch and prepare the joints involved in those upcoming motions without added risk of injury.

Cardio Training

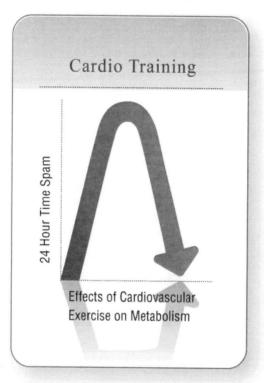

Cardio Training

24 Hour Time Spam

Effects of Cardiovascular Exercise on Metabolism

Cardiovascular (or aerobic) fitness describes the ability of the heart, lungs, and blood vessels (referred to as the cardiovascular, cardiopulmonary, or cardiorespiratory system) to deliver an adequate supply of oxygen to exercising muscles.

There are numerous ways in which to measure your cardiovascular or aerobic fitness level, including the One-Mile Walk Test, 1.5-Mile Run Test, and the Three-Minute Step Test. You can find out more on how to do these tests in the last chapter of the book, "Self-Assessment." Tracking the results of your fitness tests once a month will illustrate your progress over time. Checking your progress periodically will provide data necessary for determining the need for changes to your current workout regimen. Improved fitness test scores will also provide excitement and motivation for staying on track nutritionally and physically.

Cardiovascular exercise promotes a large number of health-related benefits, which include:

- Decreased body fat
- Decreased resting heart rate
- Decreased risk of cardiovascular disease
- Decreased risk of obesity and hypertension
- Increased energy and stamina
- Less fatigue
- Prevention and treatment of diabetes
- Decreased stress and anxiety
- Decreased risk of injuries
- Increased cardio health by strengthening the heart, its vessels, along with the circulatory and respiratory systems
- Provides a foundation for performance of all conditioning programs and sports

To determine whether an activity will promote aerobic benefits, these four guidelines must be followed:

(1) You must sustain rhythmic muscular activity, ideally using the large muscle groups, such as

legs, which will increase cardiovascular work and intensity.

(2) You must maintain a minimum of at least twenty minutes duration while exercising.

(3) You must maintain a level of exercise intensity between 60 to 80 percent of your MHR.

(4) Schedule exercise for a minimum of three days per week to maintain current health and five days per week for creating change. Ideally, for weight loss, a duration of sixty to ninety minutes of exercise is recommended five days a week.

As shown in the section regarding heart rate, there are two levels of cardiovascular conditioning. The first is the fat burning zone, and the second is the cardiovascular conditioning zone:

(1) The *fat burning zone* is reached when you are working at an effort level that is 60 to 70 percent of your MHR, as shown in the heart rate formula earlier. If your major goals are to lose weight and tone up, then incorporate more of this type of training into your program. The benefit to exercising in the fat-burning zone, especially for someone who is deconditioned (i.e., out of shape), is that they can work longer and burn more calories before fatiguing. This is especially true for a deconditioned individual, who can experience feelings of dizziness or nausea if he or she works out too hard early on in

starting a workout program. The lower intensity allows the body to burn and use fat as its main source of energy, therefore creating a leaner physique.

(2) When you're working in the *cardio zone,* your level of intensity is 70 to 80 percent of your MHR or higher. While in this zone your body needs quick energy and ultimately uses the sugar found in your blood first. You can receive benefits from higher intensity training very quickly, even if you only perform it for a few minutes at first. This type of training is also very beneficial for complementing other types of training, such as weight lifting. When you incorporate higher intensity aerobic training into your regular exercise program, it makes the other training seem easier due to the improved functioning of the heart and respiratory systems. The key is to build up to higher intensities by adding short bouts of high intensity training to your regular cardiovascular or weight training program. Over time, you can add more and more high intensity cardiovascular training to your program, resulting in faster fat losses.

High Intensity Training
is Where It's At!

While lower intensity training is great for keeping the body active and maintaining weight, people need to do high intensity training regularly. There are a lot of ways to do so, such as by taking a boot camp, running sprints or bleachers, jumping rope, and/or doing calisthenics.

What's so special about high intensity training? For one thing, high intensity training gets your internal core temperature up higher and longer for high calorie expenditure and extended fat burning after your workout. One reason most people aren't impressed by how much fat and/or weight they're losing is because they are not training at high enough intensities to get results and don't adjust their intensity once their body gets acclimated to training harder.

For even faster fat burning results and great cardiovascular improvements, try working in the anaerobic ranges of 80 to 90 percent of your max heart rate range for short bouts of thirty to ninety seconds several times during your normal workout routine. Over time, you will notice the high intensity training becomes easier, while what used to be low intensity for you becomes effortless because you've been raising the roof on your high intensity training threshold.

Weight Training

Here is why I contend that thinking fit equals being fit: if I told you that by merely adding more muscle to your body you could burn more calories simply sitting around, wouldn't you think that was the biggest exercise revolution known to man? Wouldn't you want to know more about this fat burning, metabolism-boosting, surefire "secret" to melting away the pounds?

Sure you would; there's just one little problem: this "secret" has been around for centuries and is really no secret at all. The fact of the matter is that weight training will help you burn fat by boosting your metabolism. Not only will you burn more fat faster, but you'll be less likely to get fat in the future. Now that's something even the biggest exercise-phobic can wrap his or her brain around!

Unfortunately, many people underestimate the importance of weight training in a well-balanced exercise plan. Lean muscle is the primary determinant of your body's resting metabolic rate, or RMR. RMR is the amount of energy, or calories, needed to support the various functions that go on within the body. These functions include the beating of the heart, respiration, maintenance of body temperature, and repair of bodily tissues, such as muscle and/or other cellular repair. RMR does not include calories needed for activity, such as activity related to exercise.

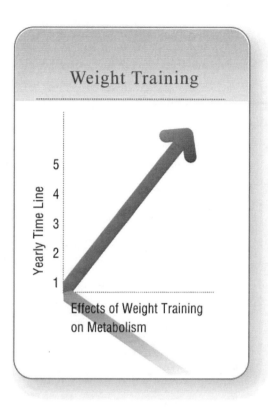

Weight Training

Yearly Time Line

5
4
3
2
1

Effects of Weight Training
on Metabolism

Your body loses approximately 2 percent of its total lean muscle per decade after the age of twenty. For a person who weighs 150 pounds and has 20 percent body fat, this means by the time he/she is age fifty he/she will be burning 216 to 360 less calories daily than when he/she was at age twenty. If that same person has had a bad habit of skipping meals, going on fad diets, eating high calorie, unhealthy foods, or starving him or herself throughout his/her life, this number can be drastically higher.

Muscle loss over time is the major contributing factor for increases in weight gain and added body fat as a person ages. You would probably agree that it was easier to lose scale weight when you were younger compared to now. This is due to the loss of muscle over the years, which caused your metabolism to slow as a result of poor nutritional habits. By adding resistance training to your program, you will increase your overall muscle mass and ultimately increase your metabolism and the number of calories you burn while doing nothing at all.

A faster running metabolism will allow you to burn fat more quickly. You will notice improvements in your physical appearance, like enhanced muscle tone and definition. These changes to your metabolism are, for the most part, permanent. Reduction in muscle mass and metabolism will only occur if you start the destructive cycle of starving and fad dieting all over again.

Injuries, improper standing or sitting habits, surgeries, overuse, and other problems we encounter over time can cause muscle imbalances. These imbalances lead to joint instability, joint wear and tear, arthritis, bone spurs, pain, disc herniations, and other musculoskeletal related problems. In fact, approximately 80 percent of all back and neck problems are preventable when a safe and effective exercise program has been specifically developed to suit a person's needs. A well-developed resistance training routine will correct imbalances that cause pain and injury. Some other positive effects that resistance training plays on the body:

- Increased muscular endurance
- Proper muscle balance
- Better posture
- Increased strength and stamina
- Increased tendon and ligament strength
- Increased joint stability, resulting in less injuries and other joint related problems
- Decreased onset of osteoporosis
- Increased joint shock absorption, resulting in less joint pain and wear and tear
- Better overall mood

CHOOSING THE RIGHT WEIGHT

Now that you understand the benefits of adding resistance training to your program, it is time to learn some fundamentals about proper resistance training. Lifting weights that are too heavy or too light, using momentum, and improper form and/or technique are common mistakes when working out with weights.

Training too heavy and using momentum is very dangerous and should be prevented. By decreasing the amount of weight and slowing down the movement to a two-second count during the positive, or concentric (muscle shortening), stage of the movement and a four-count during the negative, or eccentric (muscle elongation) stage of the movement, you will increase the intensity of your workout dramatically. This allows you to isolate specific muscle groups for maximum muscular development and the strengthening of specific groups of muscles.

Training too light is yet another common mistake that can lead to decreased results and motivation. A perfect example of this is when I see moms carrying around a thirty-pound laundry basket or forty-pound child during their day-to-day routines yet only lifting five to ten pounds at the gym. Heck, a gallon of milk weighs 8.6 pounds. One benefit of exercise is to make daily activity easier, but if you're not challenging yourself enough at the gym, then daily activity will not become easier. When you train hard, or at least at your individual strength, you get lean.

When working both too heavy and too light can hinder results, how can you determine how much weight to use when working out? The answer is to train according to your individual strength.

The easiest way to determine your individual strength is to start with a weight light enough for you perform at least twenty repetitions. Starting off with twenty reps will allow you to get a feel for the weight and allow you to maintain proper form during the movement. Next, slowly increase the weight with each set until you reach a heavy enough weight so that you can perform between twelve to fifteen reps.

The last three reps should be very difficult to accomplish, to the point that performing another repetition is almost impossible. Even though the last few reps are challenging to finish, you should be able to maintain proper form during the entirety of the motion. If you start to use incorrect form to complete the set, it is important to stop immediately to prevent injury. When you can accomplish twelve to fifteen reps and no more, then you have found the correct weight for your individual strength.

The intensity of a weight routine can also be rated between one and ten: one meaning "I could do this all day," and ten being "I cannot possibly do more." Get the picture? Obviously, either extreme is too extreme. In other words, you don't want to be doing something so easy/light that you get no benefit from it, nor do you want to do something so difficult/heavy that you hurt yourself. So where *should* you start? I recommend starting somewhere in the four to five intensity range for your first set. This is about 40 to 50 percent of your maximum strength.

If you are performing three sets of an exercise, your effort level should feel something like this:

- Set one: effort level four to five (warm-up set)
- Set two: effort level six to seven
- Set three: effort level eight to ten

An exercise routine is infinitely variable and is dependant upon the amount of time and number of days you can commit to your program. Your fitness level, personal goals, and individual needs will change over time, so add variety to your program and change things up periodically.

Cooling Down

Like warming up, cooling down is an essential part of a workout program. Unfortunately, it's one step that far too many people skip. It's understandable: you're hot, you're tired, you've got things to do, and hey, it's not like you didn't warm up, right? So what if you skip the cooling down session?

Well, warming up and cooling down are like bookends to a satisfying and safe workout. And what happens when we only use one bookend? That's right—the books fall down. Well, when you skip the cool down section of your workout, it's unfortunately only half as effective. So be smart and think twice before skipping this all-important step.

Whenever an exercise session is stopped abruptly, blood tends to accumulate or pool in an area of the body, which may cause lightheadedness. Muscle movement helps squeeze blood back toward the heart, allowing your cardiovascular system to readjust your blood flow and bring your heart rate down to normal, thus decreasing cardiac work. This ensures adequate circulation to the muscles, brain, and heart while reducing any tendencies toward fainting or dizziness.

The fitter you are, the faster your heart rate will return to normal. During this part of your program, it is important to continue with a low intensity exercise, such as aerobics, jogging, walking, cycling, or stretching to ensure proper cool down. The intensity of this activity is going to be much lighter than your actual workout, so monitor your heart rate during the cool down phase and work until it returns back to a normal resting rate. Other added benefits of cooling down properly after every workout include reduced delayed muscle soreness and stiffness; plus, this is a great time to work on flexibility improvements.

Muscle Soreness

Now here is where your mind truly can be your enemy when it comes to exercise. All our lives we're taught to avoid pain, to beware of physical harm. But what if I told you that a little pain—at least a little muscle soreness—can actually be good for you?

Now this is a long way away from your old high school coach's mantra of "no pain, no gain," but, in fact, it's entirely natural—and even beneficial—for your muscles to be sore after an extremely effective workout (In fact, I would go so far as to say be leery when you're *not* a little sore after a workout sometimes because it might mean you're not working hard enough to get results).

Muscle soreness may be felt from one to three days following exercise. Soreness is caused from microscopic tears of the muscle fibers and lactic acid production directly resulting from exercise. Although it might sound damaging, microscopic tears caused by training are actually a positive benefit of exercise because they heal and make the muscle cells larger and stronger.

Warming up before your routine and stretching afterward can help to prevent some delayed muscle soreness but not necessarily all of it. If muscle soreness is experienced, light cardiovascular exercise followed by stretching will promote healing and eliminate soreness and stiffness much more quickly.

If you have only recently begun an exercise program, it is more than likely you will experience some muscle soreness within the first few weeks of your program. If soreness persists or is accompanied by lack of range of motion (ROM), then consult your physician.

TRAINING

There are five different types of training programs that focus on specific fitness objectives:

(1) Sport specific training
(2) Fat burning training
(3) Muscle gain training
(4) Cardiovascular fitness training
(5) Flexibility training

Creating a program specific to your goals and needs can be easy once you have a basic understanding of the five varying types of training and the goals associated with each one.

Sport Specific Training

Sport specific training means exactly that: you are training to improve your conditioning related to a specific sport, such as football or golf. Ultimately this type of program has two objectives, which are improved overall fitness and enhanced sport specific skills.

Improving overall fitness will boost one's cardiovascular conditioning and flexibility, along with muscle strength and endurance. This will create general improvements that will allow an individual to play longer and harder with less fatigue.

This type of training focuses on improving sport specific skills. These skills are specific to each individual sport and focus on improving technique, form, strength, and flexibility for the sport. For instance, a soccer player may work to develop foot skills and agility for better performance on the field. You may also train to compete in an event, such as a bodybuilding competition or a triathlon. Training may be focused on other elements like timed performance, physique symmetry, or set routines.

Sport specific training usually has a varying program divided into blocks of training that may last weeks or months at a time. This type of training is called "periodization training" and usually entails blocks of time where training programs differ from one period to the next and are geared toward pre-season, on-season, post-season, and/or off-season training.

Fat Burning Training

Wouldn't it be nice if we could put on a pair of X-ray glasses, peer inside our bodies, and actually see the fat burning away from all this exercise? Unfortunately, no such glasses exist. But we do have a gauge by which we can tell whether or not we're burning fat, and it's the good old ticker.

That's right; the only way to know if you are burning fat or not is to monitor your heart rate. Many fat-loss programs include an abundance of lower intensity training because you can maintain a longer duration, which over time adds up. Keep in mind that working in the higher intensities, even for short bouts, will increase the amount of calories you burn during each workout, equating to faster weight loss.

Activities that are best for fat burning include aerobic activities, such as walking, jogging, aerobics, biking, swimming, hiking, et cetera. The key to exercising for fat burning is to make sure you are maintaining at least 60 to 70 percent of your MHR for a duration of at least twenty minutes or more. If your heart rate is lower than 60 percent of MHR, you will be working too light, and you are not going to reach your fat-loss goals, which can lead to discouragement and lack of motivation in the long run.

Consistent cardiovascular training will lead to improved conditioning; therefore, it will be necessary to increase the intensity level of your workouts in an effort to keep challenging the body. For instance, you may start a cardio program by working out three days a week on the elliptical at an intensity level of one for one full hour of training, which places your heart rate in the fat burning zone. After about four to six weeks, though, you may notice that this workout is not as difficult as it originally was and that your heart rate consistently stays below the fat burning zone. This is a sure sign that that your overall fitness level has improved and that it is time to change your program. Changing your program will ensure that you are working in the correct zone for what your goals are, which in this case is fat burning. Once again, the key to making sure you are not wasting your time in the gym is to monitor your heart rate during workouts.

Muscle Gain Training

Gaining muscle is not only for those who wish to have a bulky, sculpted physique, similar to those beastly looking men and women you see in some of the fitness magazines. Muscle building is for everyone, young and old. In fact, you might say the older you get, the more you need to be concerned about building muscle. That's because after the age of twenty you begin losing 2 percent of your lean muscle mass every decade. The problem with this trend is that your muscle is the main regulator of your metabolism. Yes, the more muscle you have, the higher your metabolism will be. For instance, a bodybuilder that weighs around 350 pounds may consume as much as ten thousand or more calories a day, just to maintain the muscle on his body. Amazing!

The reason for this amazing fact is that muscle uses energy, and the more of it you have, the more calories you burn. Think of it like an engine of a motor vehicle: the larger the engine, the more gas it uses. This concept is very much like muscle and the body. I am not suggesting by any means that you get huge or even remotely close to it. In fact, it is not possible for most people, especially women, to create two hundred to three hundred pounds of pure muscle. Women do not have testosterone like men do; therefore, they are unable to naturally get nearly as big as men.

When it comes to building muscle, however, I am suggesting that you do increase your lean muscle mass in an effort to increase your metabolic rate for higher calorie burning at rest and for creating a leaner physique. The concept of tone, or lean, really means possessing more muscle and less fat on your body than what you already have.

Muscle is denser than fat and takes up one-third of the space that fat does. In other words, one pound of fat is three times bigger than one pound of muscle. This means that if you put on ten pounds of muscle and lose ten pounds of fat, you will weigh the same on the scale, but your body will be one to two sizes smaller in clothing size.

So how do we start building this fat burning muscle? The heavier weight you lift, the more muscle you will build, and ultimately the smaller and denser your body will become. You will want do this until you build the right amount of muscle for the goals and clothing size you are trying to reach. Believe me, I weigh about 120 pounds, and there have been times in my training history that I have squatted 180 pounds, done one arm rows with 65-pound dumbbells, and bench pressed as much as 135 pounds, and I am obviously not a big girl. In fact, my normal pants size is a five, and my dress size is a small.

When I have trained for fitness competitions in the past, I have weighed as much as 125 pounds but only wore a size three in pants that were bagging off of me because my body fat was only 11 percent for the event. Now compare this to a time when I weighed 120 pounds but had a body fat of 32 percent after my son was born but wore a size seven/eight pants that were tight. Bodybuilding, or building the body healthy, is the key to creating a lean physique. It does not mean that you will look like a huge muscle-bound bodybuilder. Instead, it means that you will create the toned body you have been wanting.

If muscle weighs more than fat, does your weight really matter? No, not really. The most important thing to look at is body fat and clothing size. The less body fat you possess, the more toned your body will appear. In fact, getting *too* lean can even give the appearance of being much bigger than you really are.

Take a close, careful look at the pictures on the next page, which depict me at various weights and body fat percentages throughout my life. As you can see, it is not the weight that matters but the amount of fat that you hold on your physique.

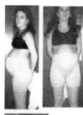

Weight: 125 lbs.
Body Fat: Pregnant (unable to test)
Pants Size: Equivalent to 11-12+ (non-maternity)

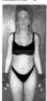

Weight: 120 lbs.
Body Fat: 32%
Lean Weight: 81.6 lbs.
Fat Weight: 38.4 lbs.
Pants Size: 7/8 extremely tight

Weight: 130 lbs.
Body Fat: 13%
Lean Weight: 113.1 lbs.
Fat Weight: 16.9 lbs.
Pants Size: 5

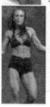 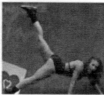

Weight: 125 lbs.
Body Fat: 11%
Lean Weight: 111.25 lbs.
Fat Weight: 13.75 lbs.
Pants Size: Size 3 was too big

Cardiovascular Fitness Training

If you are training for the health of your heart, then you are training for cardiovascular fitness. The intensity of aerobic exercise for conditioning of the heart and lungs is higher than that of cardio for fat burning; therefore, your target heart rate should be 70 to as high as 90 percent of your max heart rate.

Any aerobic activity will do, as long as you are able to maintain a higher heart rate for at least ten minutes or more. You can receive benefits from higher intensity training very quickly, even if you only perform it for a few minutes at first. This type of training is also very beneficial for complementing other types of training, such as weight lifting. When you incorporate higher intensity aerobic training into your regular exercise program, it makes the other training seem easier due to the improved functioning of the heart and respiratory systems.

If you are going to be training at higher aerobic intensities, it is important that you eat at least two hours prior to your workout. Working out in the cardio zone requires quick energy for fuel, and therefore, your body will use the glucose in your blood for this type of training first. Once all of the sugar has been burned up, you may experience hypoglycemia. Have you ever gotten sick to your stomach or lightheaded in the middle of an exercise session? Then you were probably experiencing hypoglycemia, or low blood sugar levels, either from not eating or from training too hard prior to your body's ability to do so. If this happens to you, drink some fruit juice or eat a piece of candy immediately to boost your blood sugar back to a normal level as quickly as possible in order to prevent serious repercussions.

Flexibility Training

For all those who have muscle on their body, flexibility training is for you. Yes, this means everyone. Flexibility training should be done before and after every workout, initially for warming up of soft tissues and injury prevention then later for improved flexibility. It is imperative that you always warm up your body before performing stretching.

There are two types of stretching that you should be aware of: passive and active stretching.

PASSIVE STRETCHING

Passive stretching seems to be practiced more often by most individuals than active stretching. Most likely the main reason for this is due to ignorance about the two types, how they differ, and the benefits of performing one over the other. Passive stretching encompasses the use of unrelated muscles to those being stretched, for bringing your body into further ROM in an effort to improve flexibility for those muscles being stretched.

For example, sit down on the floor with your legs together and straighten them out in front of you. Reach forward to stretch the hamstrings or back of the legs by reaching toward your toes. After you reach forward as far as you can, trying to touch your toes, grab your lower legs and pull yourself slightly farther. By grabbing your legs and using your upper body muscles to increase the intensity and ROM of your stretch, you are passively stretching. It's like lifting weights with your arms but expecting your legs to get the results. Due to the fact that you are using unrelated muscles to help you gain further motion, i.e., your upper body muscles, you may feel a deeper stretch. The problem is that you are not really affecting your flexibility in the long term.

ACTIVE STRETCHING

The second type of stretching is active stretching. Being flexible means being in balance muscularly. All muscles work together to produce movement, and they want to contract all the time. If you were to take one of your muscles out of your body and lay it on the table, it would continue to shorten to about one-third of its original length. This is what your muscles are trying to constantly do inside your body. They are pulling against the resistance of the other opposing muscles. Therefore, flexibility training really means muscle balance training. You are stretching your muscles so as to maintain balance between two opposing groups. In other words, the biceps bend your arm, and your triceps straighten your arm. By stretching regularly, you will maintain good range of motion of the joint and create a flexibility balance between the two opposing groups.

Therefore, if when you try stretching your hamstrings you instead reach forward to touch your toes and then squeeze your quadriceps and use your abs and hip flexors to pull yourself farther forward to feel a deeper stretch, you would be actively stretching. The hip flexors, quads, and abs are all playing a role for increasing your ROM during the stretch. By utilizing them to gain further mobility and feel a deeper stretch, these muscles are gaining strength and ultimately affecting your flexibility more permanently.

Using opposing muscle groups to stretch muscles, such as by squeezing the upper back muscles to feel a stretch in the chest or squeezing the triceps muscles to feel a stretch in the biceps, strengthens those muscles and therefore helps to improve strength balance and flexibility between the two groups.

Flexibility is more about strength balance between opposite groups than it is about really stretching. You can enhance overall flexibility while improving your overall muscle strength and balance between opposite muscle pairs by stretching actively instead of passively and therefore should incorporate this type of stretching into your program as your primary stretch style.

For continued improvements in flexibility, try combining stretching with a resistance or weight training program, which will help maintain muscle strength, endurance, and balance between opposing groups.

FEEL THE BURN

The beauty of fitness is that once you finally "feel the burn," that pleasant sensation of your body doing what it was meant to do, you can at last see how the mind and body work in concert. And that is when you really *will* start to *Think Fit 2 Be Fit*.

True fitness really is contagious. Why do I say "true" fitness? Because what most people do on a regular basis simply won't lead them to being fit. They work out too hard at times, not hard enough at others. They switch up, switch off, go through phases, skip workouts, make excuses, and although they may exercise two to three times per week, it's not effective or long or sincere enough to truly pay off in measurable benefits.

Hence, they never feel the burn, and they never experience what it means to truly enjoy the body as a working mechanism that can improve every other area of life as well. That is when the mind and muscle connect and when you become an exerciser for life.

Pain is never a goal regardless of your training effort; however, feeling the burn usually is. The burning sensation you may feel during exercise is a natural feeling caused by the buildup of lactic acid and increased blood flow in the working muscles. It is a natural occurrence of exercise and therefore should not raise any reasons for concern. When pain or any other discomfort is felt during exercise, double-check your form first and make any necessary adjustments in an effort to eliminate the discomfort. If pain or discomfort continues, stop immediately and consult a professional or medical doctor for investigation of the cause.

THE EXERCISE POINT SYSTEM

You made some great gains when you first started working out, but now you have hit a plateau. Why? This happens for many reasons. One reason for this is workout intensity. Your fitness level may have increased over the course of your training program, but you may have never changed the intensity of your program. Basically, the workouts have gotten easier and therefore are not challenging enough for your body to progress any further. The best way to determine if you're working hard enough is by monitoring your heart rate, but you can also use this point system to aid you in adjusting your program if you're looking to step things up and burn fat faster.

Below, I have put together a point system in an effort to help you avoid the problem of results plateau. The point system will help you determine what intensity level you should be working at for continued progress toward reaching your personal fitness and weight loss goals.

For those just starting a workout program, shoot for 5 points a week:

- Goal points per day = 1: per week = 5 points

For those who have been training for six months or longer, shoot for 10 points per week:

- Goal points per day = 2: per week = 10 points

For the advanced, shoot for 15–20 points per week:

- Goal points per day = 3–4: per week = 15–20 points

For the athlete, shoot for 20–30 points per week:
- Goal points per day = 5–6 per week = 25–30 points

Intensity / Resistance Point Chart

Points	Intensity	Training	Duration
1	Low (between 40 – 60% max HR)		
2	Moderate (60 – 75% max HR)	CARDIO	
3	High (75 – 90% max HR)		1 HOUR
1	Light (moderate weight 15 – 20 reps)		
2	Moderate weight 8 – 15 reps)	WEIGHT / RESISTANCE	
3	High (heavy weight 4 – 10 reps)		

Weight/Resistance Training Goals

Light: For those who are looking for that long, lean appearance.

Moderate: For those who are looking for a toned, more defined look and overall body reshaping.

Heavy: For those looking for more muscular development, definition, or faster results.

The purpose of the point system is to train based on intensity. If you are not training at the right intensity for your goals, then you will become disheartened over time when those goals are not attained. Over time, as your fitness level increases, your workout intensity and duration should also be increased.

To exemplify how this point system might work and what a workout might look like in real time, I have provided a sample workout on the following pages. This sample workout can be honed, modified, and, above all, personalized to fit your own intensity and duration needs.

SAMPLE WORKOUT

(1) Your exercise program is to be performed five days a week.

- Days one, three, and five will consist of the sample exercise on the following pages with your choice of high intensity callisthenic exercises in between each depicted exercise.

- Days two and four will consist of pre-breakfast, low intensity cardiovascular exercise for maximum fat burning results.

(2) Always warm up for ten to fifteen minutes each day with some low intensity aerobic activity.

(3) Weight training days

- Begin your workout performing the exercises listed on the following pages in the chronological order they are listed.

- For each exercise do one warm-up set at 50 percent of the heaviest weight you will use during your core workout phase in order to prepare the joints and connective tissues for the upcoming work.

- Perform each exercise for ten to twenty repetitions for three to four sets each.
- In between each exercise, choose a high intensity callisthenic activity to maximize fat-loss results, such as jumping jacks, burpees, jumping squats or lunges, jumping rope, wind sprints, or any other high intensity you can maintain for thirty to sixty seconds.
- Cardio day
- Perform first thing in the morning, in the fat burning zone, before you eat breakfast. Eat immediately after exercise. Use the heart rate formula mentioned earlier to determine target heart rate.

(4) When you are finished with your workout, stretch every major muscle group for thirty to sixty seconds each.

Dumbbell Chest Press to Fly on Stability Ball

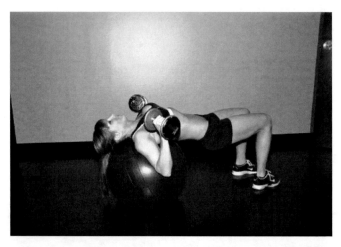

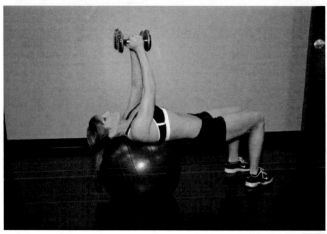

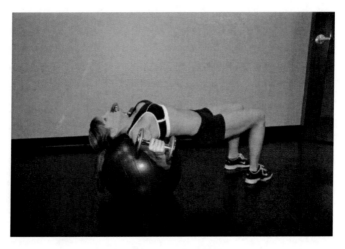

(1) Sit on the middle of the ball and then roll onto your back.

(2) Stabilize yourself with your feet on the floor about twelve to fifteen inches apart.

(3) Position dumbbells slightly outside and above your shoulders.

(4) Your palms should face toward your lower body, and your starting position should look like the starting picture.

(5) Bend your elbows at a ninety-degree angle so that your upper arms are parallel to the ground and your wrists are directly over your elbows.

(6) Press the weights up over the center of your chest in a triangular motion while simultaneously rotating your hands until the palms of your hands are facing each other above the centerline of your body, as depicted in picture two.

(7) As you lift, concentrate on keeping the weights balanced and under control.

(8) Now, while keeping the elbows locked in a slightly bent position, lower your arms toward the floor until you feel a stretch in your chest, as depicted in picture three.

(9) Exhale during the exertion phases of these movements.

(10) Repeat for a total of fifteen to twenty reps.

Wide to Narrow Squats

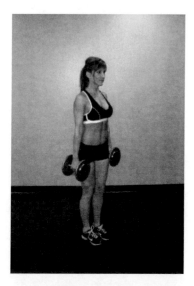

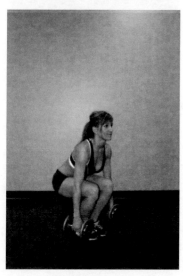

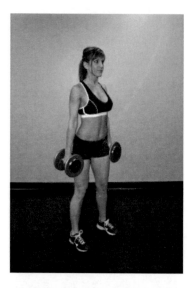

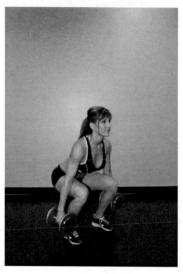

(1) Start by standing with your feet hip-width apart and the dumbbells at your sides, as depicted in picture one.

(2) During all phases of the movement, your knees should be directly in line with your ankles and perpendicular to the floor. Keep the weight of your body on your heels and not forward on your toes, and do not allow your knees to jut forward beyond your toes in the lowest position of each phase of the exercise in order to prevent strain on the knees.

(3) Slowly squat down until the tops of your thighs are parallel to the floor and your knees are bent ninety degrees, as depicted in picture two.

(4) Exhale on the way up.

(5) Step into a wider position, about shoulder-width apart, as depicted in picture three.

(6) Squat down, as depicted in picture four.

(7) Exhale as you stand up to the starting position.

(8) Repeat for a total of fifteen to twenty reps.

Switch Row

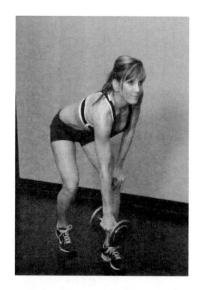

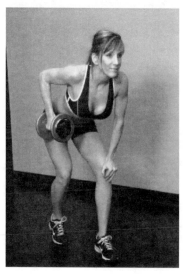

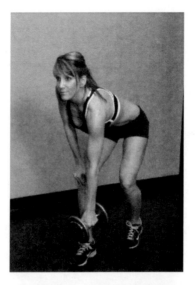

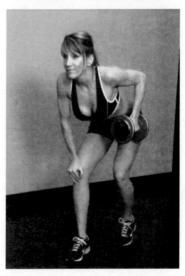

(1) Start in a bent over position, with a flat back, feet staggered front to back for stability, and your arm extended, as depicted in picture one.

(2) Exhale as you slowly pull the dumbbell up while squeezing your mid-back muscles and pulling the shoulder down and back simultaneously, as depicted in picture two.

(3) Return to the staring position.

(4) Next, turn your body forty-five degrees to the side and switch the hand that is holding the dumbbell.

(5) Repeat steps 1–4 on the other side.

(6) Repeat steps 1–5 for a total of fifteen to twenty reps each side.

Stability Ball Bicycle Crunch

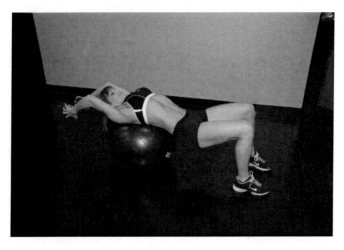

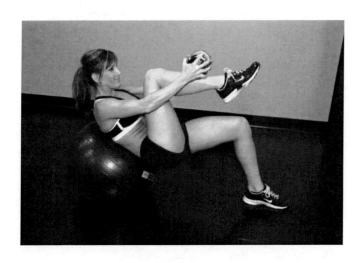

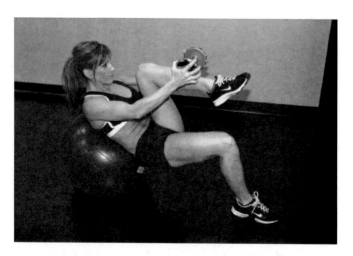

(1) Start by sitting on the ball and rolling out until your mid back is resting comfortably on the ball.

(2) Hold a dumbbell or medicine ball between your hands firmly.

(3) With the arms extended and elbows slightly bent and locked in place, raise the dumbbell over your head until you feel a stretch in your abs, as depicted in picture one.

(4) Next, pull the dumbbell slowly toward your feet while lifting one leg, as depicted in picture two.

(5) Repeat with the other leg, as depicted in picture three.

(6) Repeat steps 1–5 on each side for fifteen to twenty reps.

Around the World Bicep Curls

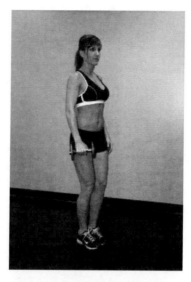

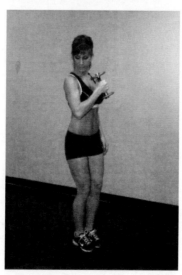

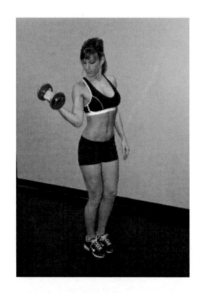

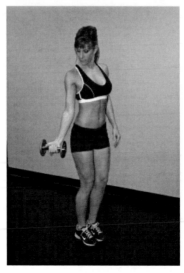

(1) Stand with the dumbbell in the starting position, as depicted in picture one.

(2) Slowly curl the dumbbell up while internally rotating the arm, as depicted in picture two.

(3) Once you reach a fully flexed position, continue the motion by externally rotating the arm while lowering the weight, as depicted in pictures three and four.

(4) Repeat for fifteen to twenty reps for each arm.

Rocking Triceps Extension

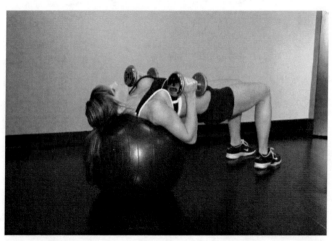

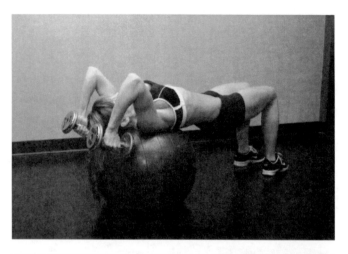

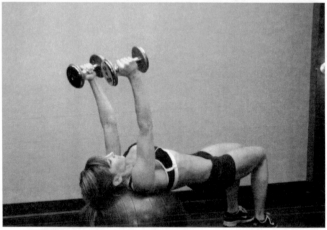

(1) Start by rolling out on the stability ball until your upper back is resting comfortably on the ball.

(2) Hold the dumbbells with your palms facing toward each other at a ninety-degree position at your sides, as depicted in picture one.

(3) Keeping the elbows bent in a ninety-degree position, raise your arms over your head until you feel a stretch in your triceps, as depicted in picture two.

(4) Next, simultaneously straighten your arms while bringing them to a position in midline with your chest, as depicted in picture three.

(5) Repeat for fifteen to twenty reps.

STEP 6:

Move to Lose

As we just discussed in step five, our bodies are designed to move. Unfortunately, now more than ever, our lives are designed to be sedentary. We may use our minds more and more often, but even as we use our brainpower, our muscle powers decline. We drive sitting down, work sitting down, meet sitting down, eat sitting down, and although we may be working "smarter," we're making it harder and harder for our bodies to function properly.

We have literally outsmarted our bodies—and put them in mortal danger of withering away. In fact, if anything is missing from our modern system of routines, ruts, and habitual behaviors, it is, sadly, movement. But now we're ready to change all that! This step is all about moving—moving for the benefit of our bodies *and* our brains. And we start, naturally, with our favorite.

EXERCISE AND THE BEAUTY OF FAT BURNING

As we have already seen, there is a long list of benefits that are a result of exercise, such as improved heart health, reduced risk of injury, increased energy and stamina, improved range of joint motion, increased flexibility, increased strength and endurance, decreased pain, improved mood, prevention of disease or dis-ease, and, last but not least, *fat burning!*

We can think and talk about fat all day, but the bottom line when it comes to fat is this: nobody likes it, everyone wants to get rid of it, and if you have too much, it is bad for your health.

A little fat might not seem like a big deal, but when it comes to fat, a little can mean a lot. Even carrying an extra eleven pounds of excess fat weight may increase your risk of developing arthritis by as much as 50 percent. When you talk about losing weight, it is the burning of body fat that is the ultimate goal here.

Fat is energy. One pound of fat equals 3,500 calories of energy. What this means is it will take 3,500 calories worth of activity to burn one pound of fat off of your body. Now if your goal is to lose ten pounds, then you will need to burn about 35,000 calories to reach that goal. If your goal is to lose one hundred pounds, then you will need to burn 350,000 calories before you reach your goal. Eek! That equates to a whole heck of a lot of moving!

We often think of weight as something that can't be controlled, but fit people practice something known as "weight management." In other words, these people know that fat *can* be managed—and now you do too. The basic principles of weight management are:

- *Weight loss:* Burn more calories than you consume, and you will lose weight.
- *Weight maintenance:* Consume the same amount of calories that you burn via RMR and activity or exercise, and you will maintain your current weight.
- *Weight gain:* Consume more calories than you burn via RMR and activity, and you will gain weight.

FAT STORAGE VERSUS FAT BURNING

Now that you know the basic principles of weight management, it's time to gain a better understanding of how fat storage compares to fat burning with regard to effort. We often marvel at how easy it is to gain weight and how hard it is to lose it. Well, it's not science fiction; it's science fact.

Do you know how *easy* is it to store fat when you eat the wrong foods? Take a look at this common list of food choices below to find out how many of your favorites it takes to store one pound of fat on your body:

- 2.25 Appetizer Samplers—Denny's
- 2.5 Deluxe Breakfasts—McDonald's
- 2.5 Nacho Mucho Grande—Taco Bell

- 3 BBQ Burgers—Denny's
- 3 Chicken Selects, 10 piece—McDonald's
- 3 32-ounce Strawberry Triple Thick Shakes—McDonald's
- 3 Chocolate Chip Cookie Dough Blizzards—Dairy Queen
- 3.5 foot-long Meatball Subs with cheese—Subway
- 5 Quarter Pounders with Cheese
- 6 large fries
- 7 blueberry muffins
- 9 pieces of German chocolate cake
- 11 cups spaghetti and meatballs (how many cups do you eat in one dinner?)
- 14 pieces of bacon
- 20 ounces of cashews

Now some of the items on this list are truly amazing. We all know that it's not that hard to eat one or two burgers—or even orders of nachos—at a fast-food restaurant. But when you think of that same meal, in one sitting, as *one pound,* it truly does stagger the mind.

Here is a list of healthy alternatives and the amount of each it would take to store a pound of fat. As you will see, it is quite difficult to store a pound of fat when you are eating healthy picks:

- 9.5 gallons broccoli
- 18 pounds of carrots
- 28 gallons of romaine lettuce

- 32 gallons of iceberg lettuce
- 33 bananas
- 44 apples
- 52 pounds of celery
- 2,187 grapes

Clearly, it is pretty easy to store one pound of fat when you are eating unhealthy food choices, but how difficult is it to *burn* that same pound of fat off your body? Each bullet point below demonstrates some general estimates of the amount of effort it will take you to burn off one pound of fat:

- 5 hours—jogging 28 miles at 5.5 miles per hour
- 6 hours—playing golf, walking, without carts
- 6 hours—biking at 10 miles per hour
- 7 hours—playing singles tennis
- 6 hours—moderate weight training
- 9.5 hours—light gardening
- 13.5 hours—child care
- 15 hours—light housework
- 15.5 hours—playing catch with a baseball
- 19 hours—laundry
- 20 hours—sex

Boy, will your house be sparkling clean and your partner happy if you accomplish burning one pound of fat with some of these means. And how many more pounds do you need to lose?

HEALTHY DIET + REGULAR EXERCISE = PERMANENT WEIGHT LOSS

As demonstrated, getting fatter is relatively simple compared to becoming leaner. That's one of the main reasons why it's so important to *Think Fit 2 Be Fit,* because if you don't have the right mind-set you will fail when it comes to these baffling and unfair odds.

There are two key strategies to permanent weight loss, and those are:

(1) Stop storing fat via healthy eating habits.
(2) Keep burning fat with regular exercise.

Many diets on the market today focus on counting calories. Unfortunately, this way of trying to lose weight only leads to failure and frustration over time. Diet after diet and year after year, people continue to count their calories and restrict the number they are eating to lose weight. This may work the first week or two, but in the end, it only destroys the body's metabolism, causing it to become slower each year.

Eating healthy alone will not get the results you desire either. You must lead an active lifestyle to burn the foods you eat on a daily basis, and you must exercise to burn the fat that is already stored on your body.

The answer to your weight loss dilemma is not that you need to eat fewer calories; consuming excessive calories is not the one and only reason why you may have gained weight in the first place. You are here today because you have not burned enough of what you have eaten to stay healthy and lean. I am not saying that you can go off the deep end and start eating as much junk food as you like as long as you burn it, because eating highly processed, fatty, and sugary foods will never help you create the body you want, no matter how much you burn. What I am saying is that it is important to make healthy dietary choices in an effort to prevent fat storage while focusing on moving more to burn the fat that is already there.

Instead of counting calories in, *count calories out.* Start by setting calorie burning goals for each week based upon the number of pounds you want to lose. Ideally, with proper diet and exercise, you can lose one-half to one and a half pounds of fat safely each week. Using these estimates and the number of calories you need to burn in order to reach your fat-loss goals that you calculated earlier in this step, determine how long it will take you to reach your goal weight on your current exercise program. Use the calorie burning charts on the following pages to determine that number.

How Long Will It Take You to Reach Your Goals?

Let's take a look at how many calories you will need to burn in excess to reach your personal weight loss goals.

Current weight _____

Desired weight _____

Pounds to lose _____

Below, multiply the number of pounds you want to lose by 3,500 calories to determine your calorie burning goals.

Pounds to lose _____ X 3,500 = _____ calories to burn

Using the activity list found on the previous pages, determine how long it will take you to reach your desired weight goals and/or percentage of body fat based on your current workout regimen. Follow the systematic process below:

Example formula:

(1) Number of exercise hours a week: 5
(2) Type of exercise: weight training free, nautilus, light/mod = 139 for thirty minutes of work
(3) 139 x 10 thirty-minute sessions = 1,390 weekly calories burned
(4) Goal weight to lose: 25 pounds
(5) 3,500 x 25 = 87,500 total calories to burn to reach weight loss goal
(6) 87,500 / 1,390 = 62 weeks to reach my weight loss goals with current routine

How long will it take you to reach your goals? Use the above example and the spaces provided below to figure out how long it will take you to reach your goals.

Number of exercise hours a week: _____

Type of exercise: _____ = _____ for thirty minutes of work

Total calories per each thirty-minute workout multiplied by number of thirty-minute workouts _____ = _____ total weekly exercise calories burned

Goal weight to lose in pounds: _____

3,500 multiplied by pounds to lose _____ = _____ total calories to burn to reach weight loss goal

Total calories to burn to reach weight loss goals _____

Divided by weekly calories burned _____ = _____ weeks to reach my weight loss goals with current routine

As you can see, you may not be burning enough calories to reach your weight loss goals in a time frame that you feel is reasonable. One way to approach this scenario is to change the type of exercise, the duration of your workouts, and/or the intensity of your current exercise regimen.

Check out the examples below:
Program One

- One hour of weight training free, nautilus, light/mod = 278 calories

Program Two

- One hour of weight training free, nautilus, vigorous = 556 calories

Program Three

- Thirty minutes of weight training free, nautilus, vigorous = 278
- Thirty minutes of jumping rope, moderate = 463
- Total calories burned in one hour = 741

By changing the type or intensity of your workouts, you can see that it is possible to burn two and a half times more calories in one workout session. This would decrease the number of weeks it would take you to reach your weight loss goals. Instead of reaching your goal in sixty-two weeks with your current exercise program, as shown in the above example, it would only take you twenty-four weeks.

What if I told you that you could get to the same destination but in half the time? You'd buy that ticket, wouldn't you? Well, that's what happens when you simply apply a little mind power to your workouts by changing the type or intensity every time you exercise.

Try applying the formulas above to determine how long it will take you to reach your goals both using your current routine and with an alternate routine that causes you to burn more calories in the same amount of time. Track the calories you burn each week to keep you on track toward reaching your fat burning goals. Use the

Calorie Tracking Sheet at the end of this chapter to keep track of your calorie expenditure.

SMALL CHANGES YOU CAN LIVE WITH

We always want the big win; we never settle for anything less than the grand prize. But when it comes to moving your body, less really *is* more. Focus on small changes that are easy to live with. Incorporate lots of activities that will increase the number of calories you are burning on a regular basis, like:

- Walking the dog two to three times a day
- Taking stairs
- Parking farther away
- Mall walking
- Walking for part of your lunch break
- Exercise while watching TV
- Eating breakfast (skipping meals slows metabolism)
- Playing with kids (kill two birds with one stone; bond with your family and stay in shape)
- Yard work
- Washing the car
- Go dancing (it is fun and you burn so many calories)

The best way to wrap your mind around moving far is to think in terms of "small things are better than *no* things." Think of how often we choose to sit rather than stand each week, to flip channels instead of hit a ball, to stay inside rather than take a walk, to drive instead of pedal a bike. If you simply add just one or two small things to every single day, you *will* get *big* results.

Making small changes that are easy to live with will get you the permanent weight loss results you are looking for. Did you know the average weight gain for adults is 1.8 pounds each year? Small incremental increases in weight are what lead to overweight and obesity in time. Each infinitesimal increase goes unnoticed, but when you continue to add 1.8 pounds of fat to your body year after year, the results are astounding. In ten years, you're eighteen pounds overweight; in twenty years, you're thirty-six pounds overweight; in thirty years, you're fifty-four pounds overweight; and so on and so forth.

Did you also know that it only takes an excess of fifteen calories a day to cause this weight gain in the first place? Yep, only fifteen calories; talk about minuscule! So when I tell you to make small changes, believe me, it does not take much to create tremendous change in your life over time.

I am sure you would agree with me when I tell you that starting off with a fifteen calorie decrease in your diet each day and burning more calories with exercise every day is not only doable; it is easy to live with and incorporate permanently into your health-driven lifestyle. Start today by making a few small changes to your workout and nutritional plan to ensure permanent weight loss success. What have you got to lose?

Oh, that's right: only fat!

HITTING A PLATEAU

Did you have great results in the beginning of your workout program but now you have hit a plateau? Now is not the time to give up; now is the time to *change things up.* Think about it: you do not stay in first grade forever, do you? No, you learn what you need to and move on to the next grade, which teaches you more and expands your way of thinking. Well, your body works in a similar fashion. When you start working out, it may be challenging, but over time, as your body adapts to exercise, the same routine becomes easier and less challenging.

A research study from the Human Performance Laboratory at Ball State University showed that periodizing (i.e., changing your program on a periodic basis) your workouts produces better results. The results of this twelve-week study, published in the journal *Medicine & Science in Sports & Exercise,* showed results of more than double in percentage of fat loss and lean muscle gained in pounds for those individuals that periodized their workouts, compared to those that did not.

Insanity is defined as doing the same thing over and over but expecting different results. If you have not changed your routine and it has been over six to twelve weeks since you started it and you are not experiencing any further progression toward your goals, then, quite frankly, you are acting "insane" (according to this definition). In other words, you are not thinking fit to be fit; you're not actually thinking fit at all.

We can't just put our workouts in a box and leave them there; we can't just check them off our to-do list and suffer through them without sweating, increasing intensity, or even switching things up from time to time.

If you want continued progress, then continue challenging your body to create those results. Changing up the type of exercise, the duration of your workout, and/or exercise intensity will shock your system and promote balanced fitness, as well as expedite change. It is recommended that you change your routine approximately every four to twelve weeks. How will you know when the time is right for a change? Use your progress to determine when it is time to make changes to your program.

If you continue to make improvements, then maintain your current routine. On the other hand, if you hit a plateau, it is a sign that it is time for a change to stimulate results once again. Changing things up will not only encourage progress; it will also prevent boredom or monotony from setting in and create an all around well-balanced healthy body.

Here are a few examples of how you can change your program in order to surprise your body and encourage continued advancements in your overall fitness.

Period One

- Weight training three days a week
    - Three sets for fifteen to twenty reps
    - One hour

- Light cardio two days a week
    - Fat burning zone
    - Thirty minutes

Period Two

- Weight training five days a week
  - ° Three sets for fifteen to twenty reps
  - ° One hour
- Light cardio two days a week
  - ° Fat burning zone
  - ° Thirty minutes

Period Three

- Weight training three days a week
  - ° Four to five sets for eight to ten reps—adjust weight accordingly
  - ° One hour
- Moderate cardio two days a week
  - ° Fat burning zone
  - ° Thirty minutes

Period Four

- Cardio five days a week for one hour
  - ° Two and a half days fat burning zone
  - ° Two and a half days cardio zone, including sprint work, jumping rope, high intensity cardio or kickboxing, et cetera

PARTING WORDS ABOUT MOVE TO LOSE

The best part about moving to lose is that you don't have to move mountains, do steroids, bench press a truck, or run a marathon to see big gains in your weight- and fat-loss goals. In fact, it doesn't take an enormous amount of effort to change your life, but it does take three simple things: *effort, thought,* and *planning.* Once again, make small changes you can live with over time, and the results will pay off in the end.

Over the last several chapters, you have learned an immense amount of information from this program, and I know it can sometimes be overwhelming once you are off on your own. In the next step we will review ways to evaluate your current program and establish the next steps in mapping your plan. You will learn to identify when your program is out of balance and how to reestablish that balance for continued success.

Tracking Calories Burned

Day	Activity	Duration	Total Calories Burned	Daily Burn Goal
Monday				
Tuesday				
Wednesday				
Thursday				
Friday				
Saturday				
Sunday				
TOTAL				

Exercise	Calories for 30 Minutes
• Aerobics class, high impact	292
• Aerobics class, low impact	208
• Aerobics class, step, with 6–8 inch step	354
• Aerobics class, water	333
• Archery, general	146
• Backpack, general	292
• Backpack with 10–20 pound load	312
• Badminton, competitive	292
• Badminton, singles and doubles	187
• Baseball, fast or slow pitch	208
• Baseball, throw/catch	104
• Basketball, shooting baskets	187
• Basketball, wheelchair	271
• Bike 16–19 mph, very fast	500
• Bike < 10 mph, leisure	167
• Bike, BMX or mountain	354
• Bike, stationary, 150 watts	292
• Bike, stationary, 50 watts	125
• Boating, power boat	104
• Bowling, lanes	125
• Boxing, punching bag	250
• Boxing, sparring	375
• Calisthenics, back exercises	146
• Calisthenics, pull-ups or jumping jacks	333
• Calisthenics, pushups or sit-ups	333
• Canoe 2–3.9 mph, light	125
• Canoe > 6 mph, vigorous	500
• Child care standing, light	117
• Child care walk/run, vigorous	208

- Circuit training, general · 333
- Clean gutter, general · 208
- Clean, heavy (windows, mop) · 125
- Clean, light (dust, vacuum) · 104
- Dance: ballroom, slow (waltz, foxtrot) · 125
- Dance: country, line, square · 187
- Dance: tango, mamba, cha-cha · 125
- Fencing, general · 250
- Fish, boat/sitting · 104
- Football, competitive · 375
- Football, flag or touch · 333
- Football, throw/catch · 104
- Frisbee, general · 125
- Garden, general · 167
- Garden, rake · 167
- Golf driving range, miniature · 125
- Golf, power cart · 146
- Golf, pull clubs · 179
- Golf, carry clubs · 208
- Gymnastics, general · 185
- Handball, general · 556
- Handball, team · 370
- Hang gliding, general · 162
- Ice skate, general · 324
- Jog, general · 324
- Jog, jog/walk combination · 278
- Jog, water · 370
- Juggling, general · 185
- Jump rope, fast · 556
- Jump rope, mod · 463

- Jump rope, slow — 370
- Kayaking, general — 231
- Kickball, general — 324
- Lacrosse, general — 370
- Laundry, general — 93
- Martial arts, judo — 463
- Martial arts, kickboxing — 463
- Martial arts, tae kwon do — 463
- Martial arts, tai chi — 185
- Motocross, general — 185
- Move furniture, carry boxes — 278
- Mow lawn: power mower, walk — 255
- Mow lawn: riding mower — 116
- Ping-pong, general — 185
- Polo, general — 370
- Racquetball, casual — 324
- Rock climb, general — 370
- Rower: stationary, 50 watts, light — 162
- Run 5 mph, 12 min/mi — 370
- Run 6 mph, 10 min/mi — 463
- Run 7 mph, 8.5 min/mi — 532
- Sailing, casual — 139
- Scrub floors, bathroom, bathtub — 176
- Sex, light (kiss, hug) — 46
- Sex, mod — 60
- Sex, vigorous — 69
- Shovel snow, hand — 278
- Ski, downhill light — 231
- Ski, downhill moderate — 278
- Swim laps freestyle, fast — 463

- Swim laps freestyle, slow/mod   324
- Tennis, doubles   278
- Tennis, singles   370
- Trampoline, general   162
- Treadmill, walk 3 mph, 20 min/mi, 0% inc   153
- Treadmill, walk 4 mph, 15 min/mi, 0% inc   231
- Volleyball, noncompetitive   139
- Walk 3 mph, 20 min/mi   153
- Walk 4 mph, 15 min/mi   231
- Walk < 2 mph   93
- Walk, push stroller   116
- Wash and wax car, boat   208
- Weight training free, nautilus, light/mod   139
- Weight training free, nautilus, vigorous   278

STEP 7:

Balance Is Key

Losing weight is big business nowadays, and some companies are making millions by selling weight loss products that prey on an individual's desire to get fit. The truth is there is no miracle pill or gadget that can help you to lose weight and get in shape permanently. If you want to lose weight for good, you need to start by addressing the root of the problem.

What would that be? The root of the problem is that your life is *out of balance.* Balance is the key to everything. A balanced physiology equates to health and vitality of the body. A balanced mind equates to mental clarity and positive thinking.

Think about it: when your checkbook is balanced, you spend more wisely. When your tires are balanced, the drive to work is smoother. Well, your body is no different; when you find balance between all those vital areas in your life—work, health, home, weight—you literally live better.

LIFE'S A BALANCING ACT

Balanced emotions equate to feelings of euphoria, love, joy, and happiness. And a balanced spirit equates to feelings of excitement and appreciation for life. Proper nutrition and exercise, along with rest and recovery, promote balance in all of these areas. If one area is imbalanced, on the other hand, then all areas are affected and thrown out of balance.

For instance, if you are not eating foods that give your body the nutrients it needs for sustained energy, you will feel tired physically, emotionally, mentally, and spiritually. We all know how we feel after a cheat weekend when we've been eating through drive-thru windows for breakfast and lunch and take-out menus for dinner and dessert. How do we feel? In a word, crappy!

And it's no wonder: fake food is no food at all. Well, when you eat junk food, fake food, frozen food, zapped food, fried food, processed food, and the like, it's kind of like you're not really eating real food at all.

Think about it: how would you feel if you did not eat for an entire day? You would feel tired, lethargic, and unmotivated, right? You might even feel irritable or stressed out. When you are tired physically, your emotions experience more negative moods, your willpower becomes weakened, and in many cases when this happens, you often make poor decisions that you would usually not make. These decisions affect your health negatively, like eating cookies due to emotional distress. These less than desirable choices are much easier to make when you are run down and tired from a long day at work or from skipping meals.

Skipping workouts leads to increased irritability, stress, lack of motivation, and low energy. Feelings of fatigue lead to more negative choices due to lack of willpower in relation to low energy levels. The destructive circle goes round and round, moving you further away from reaching your goals.

It is this type of cycle of imbalance that has brought you to where you are today. Interestingly enough, just one day of poor eating or skipping meals can generate imbalances in all other areas of your well-being. Improper eating not only affects your body but your emotional state (heart), your drive and motivation (soul), and your mental attitude (mind).

Holistic medicine teaches us that to truly be healthy it is imperative to attain balance in four areas of your life, and those areas include the heart, soul, body, and mind. Whole health means balance in every area that makes you who you are. Step seven focuses on identifying imbalances related to these four components, which, in turn, may be the primary cause of your weight gain and declining health over the years.

Recognizing your shortcomings will give you the ability to create a plan that promotes positive and proactive choices that focus on well-being. Instituting balance in your life will help to eliminate symptoms of overweight, obesity, or other health-related problems that you may be experiencing today. Remember that the issues surrounding being overweight and even potential obesity are not diseases but a "dis-ease," or imbalance of your whole self. Once balance is reestablished, the symptoms will fade away, leaving only health and vitality as the end result.

One of the main things I try to teach people is that we are a society that uses linear thinking to solve problems, but health and other problems surrounding imbalance do not usually equate to the one problem and one solution model that most off-the-shelf fitness programs and books offer.

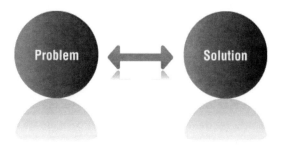

When a person is out of balance and is having weight or health issues, it is almost always if not always the result of many behaviors that created this one major problem. Therefore, it's important to understand that the problem-solution model looks more like an asterisk symbol rather that a linear model, as depicted here in the graphics.

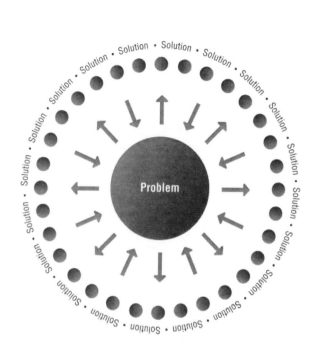

Therefore, in order to find where you are falling short, it is important to look at all areas that create whole health, ask yourself a lot of questions, answer those questions honestly, and then fill in the Wheel of Success and Wall of Despair to find what your asterisk symbol looks like and which of the many areas you may need improvement in.

With that message in mind, take a look at your current lifestyle trends to determine the areas of greatest need. You will notice that the chart below is broken down into those four major categories that create a healthy and whole you. Only a whole being can have true vitality, and with health comes the absence or elimination of dis-ease and its related ailments. Using the chart below, rate yourself to determine which areas need the most attention for you to make progress in attaining a balanced life.

Rating

	Excellent	Good	Average	Below Average	Poor
Heart					
Do you possess a sense of accomplishment when you've eaten well or exercised regularly?	Always	Most of the time	Sometimes	Rarely	Never
Do you handle stressful situations calmly and collectively?	Always	Most of the time	Sometimes	Rarely	Never
Do you use healthy activities to reduce stress in your life, instead of food?	Always	Most of the time	Sometimes	Rarely	Never
When you feel sad, do you participate in fun activities or try connecting with friends to raise your spirits?	Always	Most of the time	Sometimes	Rarely	Never
Do you feel your life is filled with joy and happiness?	Always	Most of the time	Sometimes	Rarely	Never
On the days you feel frazzled, anxious, and overwhelmed, do you workout to get rid of those unhealthy energies instead of choosing inactivity?	Always	Most of the time	Sometimes	Rarely	Never
Does your home environment give you a sense of emotional support for living healthy?	Always	Most of the time	Sometimes	Rarely	Never
Is your work life emotionally supportive for living a healthy lifestyle?	Always	Most of the time	Sometimes	Rarely	Never
Do you make time for friends and family regularly?	Always	Most of the time	Sometimes	Rarely	Never
When hanging out with friends or family, do you choose healthy activities instead of food or alcohol as your main choice of entertainment?	Always	Most of the time	Sometimes	Rarely	Never
When you do something for you, do you appreciate yourself for doing so, instead of feeling guilty?	Always	Most of the time	Sometimes	Rarely	Never

Rating	Excellent	Good	Average	Below Average	Poor
			Soul		
Do you possess a sense of accomplishment when you've eaten well or exercised regularly?	Always	Most of the time	Sometimes	Rarely	Not at all
Do you have the drive and motivation to be as healthy as you can be?	Always	Most of the time	Sometimes	Rarely	Not at all
Do you have a childlike curiosity about life and a yearning to learn more, grow more, and become a better and healthier you?	Always	Most of the time	Sometimes	Rarely	Not at all
Do you feel that you have an internal fire, drive, and excitement for living life to the fullest?	Always	Most of the time	Sometimes	Rarely	Not at all
Do you make time to do the things you love most?	Always	Most of the time	Sometimes	Rarely	Not at all
Do you take the time to connect with others that are working towards the same goals, by giving each other support and encouragement?	Always	Most of the time	Sometimes	Rarely	Not at all
Do you have a sense of purpose and/or contribution in your life?	Always	Most of the time	Sometimes	Rarely	Not at all
Imagine your life is a blank canvas. Do you feel that you are the artist, which is creating the beautiful piece of art with each day that passes and each choice you make?	Always	Most of the time	Sometimes	Rarely	Not at all
Do you have feelings of calm and centeredness?	Always	Most of the time	Sometimes	Rarely	Not at all
Do you regularly partake in activities that make you feel alive and invigorated?	Always	Most of the time	Sometimes	Rarely	Not at all

Rating	Excellent	Good	Average	Below Average	Poor
Body / Nutrition					
Do you feel that you have a well-balanced Nutritional program?	Yes		Maybe	No	
How many servings of fruits and vegetables do you eat a day?	5+	4	3	2	0 – 1
How many glasses of water do you drink a day?	8+	6 – 7	4 – 5	2 – 3	0 – 1
Do you eat only whole grain foods?	Always	Most of the time	Sometimes	Rarely	Not at all
Do you eat 2 – 4 servings of high quality protein each day?	Always	Most of the time	Sometimes	Rarely	Not at all
Do you eat mostly 1 ingredient fresh foods?	Always	Most of the time	Sometimes	Rarely	Not at all
Do you eat macronutrients based on the time of day your body needs certain foods most, as demonstrated in the food timing charts?	Always	Most of the time	Sometimes	Rarely	Not at all
How many glasses of alcohol do you consume a week?	0	1	2	3	4+
How many cups of coffee do you drink a day?	0	1	2	3	4+

Rating	Excellent	Good	Average	Below Average	Poor
Exercise & Physical Activity					
How many days a week do you exercise?	5	4	3	2	1
How many minutes do you exercise during your workouts?	90	60	30	15	0
Are you stretching before and/or after each workout?	Always		Sometimes	Never	
How many days a week do you weight train?	5	4	3	2	0 – 1
How many days a week do you do aerobic activity?	5	4	3	2	0 – 1
Are you monitoring your heart rate during exercise?	Yes		No		
What exercise intensity are you training at (refer to weight / resistance point chart)	3		2	1	
Approximately how many calories are you burning during each workout?	601+	401 – 600	201 – 400	101 – 200	0 – 100
How often do you change your workouts?	Every Month	Every 12 weeks	Once or twice year	Seldom	Never

Rating	Excellent	Good	Average	Below Average	Poor
Fitness Assessment Results					
Sit and Reach Test	Excellent	Good	Average	Below Average	Poor
Walk, Run or Step Test – Cardiovascular Health	Excellent	Good	Average	Below Average	Poor
Body Fat	Excellent	Good	Average	Below Average	Poor
BMI	Excellent	Good	Average	Below Average	Poor
Push-Up Test – Muscle Strength	Excellent	Good	Average	Below Average	Poor
Crunch Test – Muscle Endurance	Excellent	Good	Average	Below Average	Poor
Waist to Hip Ratio	Excellent	Good	Average	Below Average	Poor

Rating	Excellent	Good	Average	Below Average	Poor
Mind					
Are you a positive thinker?	Always	Most of the time	Sometimes	Rarely	Not at all
Do you possess mental clarity?	Always	Most of the time	Sometimes	Rarely	Not at all
Is your mind absent of worry and anxious thoughts?	Always	Most of the time	Sometimes	Rarely	Not at all
Is your internal dialog supportive, loving, appreciative, and kind, when thinking about yourself?	Always	Most of the time	Sometimes	Rarely	Not at all
Do you set nutrition, exercise and/or wellness goals?	Always	Most of the time	Sometimes	Rarely	Not at all
Do you reach the goals you set?	Always	Most of the time	Sometimes	Rarely	Not at all
Do you track, monitor, and update your wellness goals or progress?	Always	Most of the time	Sometimes	Rarely	Not at all
Do you think about health daily?	Always	Most of the time	Sometimes	Rarely	Not at all
Do you picture yourself fit and healthy in your own mind's eye?	Always	Most of the time	Sometimes	Rarely	Not at all
Do you read daily about fitness and living a healthy lifestyle?	Always	Most of the time	Sometimes	Rarely	Not at all

THE WHEEL OF PROGRESS
AND THE WALL OF DESPAIR

This next step involves an exercise that will clarify the areas of your life that need the most improvement. I call this exercise the Wheel of Progress. As mentioned earlier in this series of steps, compounding small and daily proactive behaviors on top of each other can lead to massive change and rewards. You don't *have* to lift the most weights, run the fastest, or come in first every day; small things, every day, help win big rewards. The more positive and proactive actions you make, the more momentum you will gain, and the faster you will reach your goals. Motivation gets you going, but habits keep you going by creating momentum.

For this exercise, you will need to count all of the proactive answers you selected for each question on the previous pages that are shaded in gray. You will then color in a block for each one under the category in which it falls.

For example, if you fell under the excellent rating for positive thinking, color in one block of the mind category on your Wheel of Progress. The goal is to have a uniformly balanced circle. Here's the reason why. Imagine that your life is that wheel: when the wheel is small, it takes longer for you to reach your destination. If the wheel is uneven, your ride is bumpy and uncomfortable. If the wheel is too imbalanced, you may try with all your might but find you have not moved from your current spot because of your wheel's unevenness.

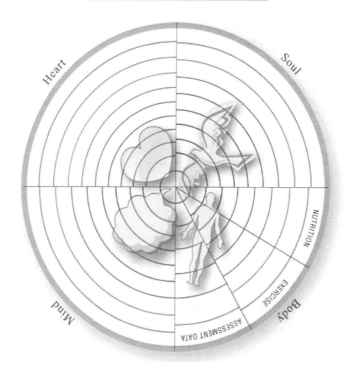

Your next exercise is to determine what actions are prohibiting your progress. I call this exercise the Wall of Despair. If you are not reaching your goals, it is because there are obstacles, which can create a wall that blocks growth.

To determine how big your wall is, count all of your selections that are not shaded in gray. For each one, fill in one brick on the Wall of Despair. The bigger your wall, the more difficulty you will have reaching your goals and the achievement of permanent weight loss.

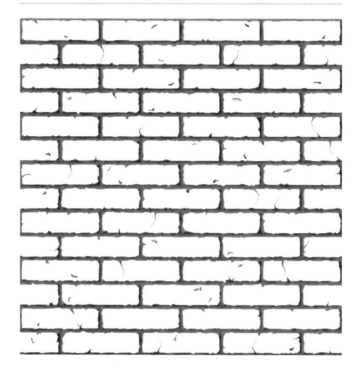

The objective of these two exercises is to help you become more aware of your behaviors and to increase your awareness of the facts of whether those choices are blocking or producing results. Your goal will be to eliminate bricks from the wall of despair by changing old, unhealthy habits to new, healthy ones. As you alter your lifestyle and improve the less than good to excellent behaviors, you will move those under-producing habits from the Wall of Despair to the Wheel of Progress.

The larger the Wheel of Progress becomes, the more speed and momentum it will pick up. Motivation gets you going, habits keep you going, and the more proactive habits you acquire, the more power you have behind generating results and success. Your wheel is comprised of small, attainable habits that when compounded create a powerful driving force to initiate change.

The larger the wheel, the less revolutions and effort it will take for you to create change. This is the reason why those individuals that are successful remain successful, because they have so much momentum and power behind their lifestyle and habits it is impossible for them not to succeed.

SUMMING IT UP

Over the course of this book, you have learned about the various components that create a well-balanced program, which, in turn, creates a well-balanced being. The key to long-term success is to take baby steps or make small, attainable changes that over time compound and create momentum, drive, and therefore outcome-driven results. Reevaluate, adjust, and fine-tune your program every four to six weeks, and this will ensure lasting change.

Living healthfully means developing the ability to effectively manage life's hectic pace by practicing behaviors that are important to your overall health. The more you juggle, the harder it becomes to maintain balance and overall health. Try simplifying your life by narrowing your focus toward immediately changing those areas that are most critically out of balance. Try choosing one or two areas in which to improve upon each month.

Reevaluate your goals on a monthly basis in an effort to make continued progress. Start this process now by choosing one to two areas to improve upon and jot down your choices on the lines below. Now, choose three small goals that will help you grow positively in those areas. Next, write three immediate actions that will expedite the process.

THREE AREAS TO IMPROVE UPON:

(1) _____

(2) _____

(3) _____

THREE GOALS TO HELP YOU ACCOMPLISH THIS:

(1) _____

(2) _____

(3) _____

THREE IMMEDIATE ACTIONS THAT WILL HELP YOU REACH YOUR GOALS:

(1) _____

(2) _____

(3) _____

Don't just do this once and call it quits. Remember to do this each and every month. This will keep you moving in the right direction. Human beings are creatures of habit and change is difficult, but with each step you take, it becomes easier due to the momentum being generated.

With every step, attaining your goals becomes more of a reality, and by practicing patience, perseverance, determination, and visualizing a clear picture of what it is that you want, you will not only make your goals a reality; you will finally gain control of your weight and health for good.

Finally, remember that balance is not some touchy-feely, New Age mumbo jumbo. Every fit person I know, every person I know who is trying to get fit, every one of my (successful) clients and gym members seeks balance because that is when they truly *Think Fit 2 Be Fit*.

THE THINK FIT 2 BE FIT ACTION PLAN:

Self-Assessment

Now that I've given you a new way to conceive your body, I want to give you a new way to *think* about your body in the first place. For many of us, what we weigh, how tall we are, even things like girth, torso, and our body mass index (or BMI) are complete mysteries.

They aren't mysteries because we aren't smart enough to figure them out or because we don't care; they're mysteries because we simply don't want to know. It's enough for us to grab a certain size off the rack, rush to the register, race home, and cut off the tag so no one knows we're a size or two bigger than we were last year, last month, or even last week.

Instead of truly assessing our current physical condition, we complain about it, lament it to friends, trouble over it, and eventually obsess about it. And the stronger an obsession gets, the harder and harder it becomes to face the truth.

Self? Meet truth! In this somewhat unpleasant but absolutely necessary chapter, I want you to start thinking differently about where you are right now because, quite simply, you have to start somewhere.

No one is here to judge; it is what it is, and the only thing you can do about the past is to face it and start moving steadily toward the future. This chapter about assessing yourself may seem daunting at first, but I guarantee you that by the time you're done you will have had a watershed moment in your life.

Why? Because you will have finally faced the truth about where you are, physically speaking, and where you need to go. Monitoring your progress is an essential step toward reaching your health and fitness goals. It allows you to create a starting point from which to set your personal standards and goals. It is vital to start with a non-biased point of reference to determine whether you are making progress or not.

Monitoring your progress can provide you with the encouragement and motivation you need to continue working toward your goals. Before you go any further, you will need to assess your overall fitness level using the instructions on the following pages.

At home or in the gym, perform the following assessments to determine your point of reference for body composition, girth measurements, waist-to-hip ratio, heart health, flexibility, as well as muscle strength and endurance.

After completing the full eight segments in this program, it is imperative that you reassess yourself on a monthly basis to continue monitoring your fitness level, which will ensure continued success and provide motivation along the way.

The good news is that these original assessments are much more rigid, controlled, and specific than those you'll continue to do throughout your own personalized program. Everyone has their own personalized way of "checking in" on their progress from time to time; most *don't* involve calipers and heavy machinery!

For instance, with myself, I know that my body fat is where it's supposed to be when I see the top two blocks of my abs, or that my cardio fitness is at a healthy place when I can run two miles consistently without stopping.

The important thing is to recognize the various cues your body sends you when things aren't going so well or you're slipping off the program. For instance, maybe for you, it will be that your new, one size smaller pants don't fit as loosely anymore, or for your neighbor, it might be that she's getting winded toward her last quarter mile.

It's important to pay attention to these cues so that you can not only reassess yourself when things aren't going as well as you'd like but also so you can first reward your positive accomplishments and then readjust to avoid a plateau in your program.

BODY COMPOSITION

An assessment of body composition will determine your actual percentage of lean body mass to body fat ratio. It can be very common for an exerciser to lose fat and gain muscle without experiencing any change in total body weight. For someone who is trying to lose weight, this can be frustrating. We feel like just because we're not getting any smaller, we're just not getting any healthier either. Also, oftentimes, a person will go down in clothing size and not be losing weight on the scale, which is even more common at first, due to the fat and muscle changes. That's why knowing your measurements gives your mind the tools it needs to feel good about your progress, to *Think Fit 2 Be Fit.*

You can have your body composition done at most local gyms or by purchasing an electrical impedance tool, which now are commonly built into many electronic scales for your home that are used to assess body fat.

Body Fat Assessment

Standard Values For % Of Body Fat

Men

Age	20–29	30–39	40–49	50–59	60+
Excellent	<10	<11	<13	<14	<15
Good	11–13	12–14	14–16	15–17	16–18
Average	14–20	15–21	17–23	18–24	19–25
Fair	21–23	22–24	24–26	25–27	26–28
Poor	>24	>25	>27	>28	>29

Women

Age	20–29	30–39	40–49	50–59	60+
Excellent	<15	<16	<17	<18	<19
Good	16–19	17–20	18–21	19–22	20–23
Average	20–28	21–29	22–30	23–31	24–32
Fair	29–31	30–32	31–33	32–34	33–35
Poor	>32	>33	>34	>35	>36

Body Fat _____

Girth Measurements

Girth measurements are measurements taken at precise locations on your body that can be used as a valuable tool in monitoring your progress. They may be used alone or in combination with skin-fold measurements for determining body fat percentage.

You may not see drastic changes in scale weight for the first three to eight weeks of the *Think Fit 2 Be Fit* program due to body composition changes. If you have dieted throughout your lifetime, you may actually lose fat and gain muscle at the same rate, therefore, causing little to no changes in body weight as measured by a scale. This is why girth measurements can be a useful tool for determining your progress.

List your girth measurements in the spaces provided below.

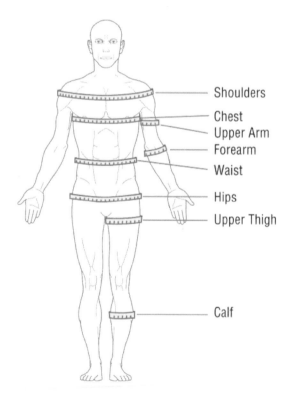

(1) Neck _____
(2) Shoulders _____
(3) Chest _____
(4) Waist _____
(5) Hips _____
(6) Thigh _____
(7) Calf _____
(8) Bicep _____
(9) Flexed Bicep _____

Girth measurements are also important for use in assessing waist-to-hip ratio. Your waist-to-hip ratio is an important tool that can help to determine your overall health risks. People with more weight or body fat stored around their stomach and waist (an apple shape) are at greater risk of lifestyle-related diseases, such as heart disease and diabetes, than those with weight or body fat stored around their hips, buttocks, and thighs (a pear shape). It is a simple and useful measurement of fat distribution.

Health Risk	Male	Female
Low Risk	0.95 or below	0.80 or below
Moderate Risk	0.96 – 1.0	0.81 – 0.85
High Risk	1.0+	0.85+

HEART HEALTH

Monitoring your pulse is important for determining heart rate and rhythm, which is caused by the beating—or pumping—of the heart. We describe the heart in terms of its rate, which is the number of beats per minute (bpm) it pumps. A fast rate can be a sign of a deconditioned heart, which usually occurs from lack of cardiovascular conditioning or exercise. When your heart rate is fast, it means that the heart is working harder to pump blood through the body.

A deconditioned heart needs to beat two to three times more often than a healthy, conditioned heart. If your heart is conditioned, it means it is stronger and can pump more blood in one pump than what an unhealthy heart can do. Think of it like this: Imagine that you and a friend are walking a two-mile path. Your friend can take really long strides at a somewhat leisurely pace, but you only get to take steps that are no more than five inches in length. Your objective is to keep up with your friend so that you reach your destination at the same time. Who do you think will tire first? You will, because you have to take many more steps then your friend while working faster to keep up.

This is exactly what your body is doing with reference to a conditioned or deconditioned heart. Blood needs to circulate through the body quickly to ensure health of all of your bodily tissues. A healthy heart pumps so hard that it forces more blood to move throughout your body with one pump than one pump of a deconditioned heart. Therefore, the deconditioned heart has to work harder and faster to get the same volume of blood to circulate to all your body's tissues.

Resting Pulse—Sixty Seconds

Resting Pulse

Age or Fitness Level	Beats Per Minute (bpm)
Babies to age 1	100–160
Children ages 1 to 10	60–140
Children age 10+ and adults	60–100
Well-conditioned athletes	40–60

Use the instructions below to assess your resting pulse and to determine your heart rate.

- Purpose: To evaluate the heart's resting heart rate by monitoring the number of times it beats in a minute.
- Equipment needed: Watch with second hand.

Directions:

- Measure your resting pulse in the morning before getting out of bed or partaking in any activity.
- Take your pulse at the wrist or neck. It will probably be between fifty and one hundred beats per minute (bpm).
- Wrist pulse: Place two fingers just below the base of the thumb and to the center of your arm.

- Neck pulse: Place two fingers halfway between the windpipe and the muscle at the side of the neck.
- Count the number of times your pulse or heart beats for one full minute and record.
- Repeat three days in a row and record.
- Add the three days of resting heart rates and divide by three for an average resting heart rate.
- Resting Heart Rate: _____ bpm

Recovery Heart Rate

Recovery heart rate assesses the health of your heart when placed under stress. The faster your heart rate returns to normal, the better the score and the more conditioned your heart is. Choose one recovery heart rate test—the One-Mile Walk Test, the 1.5-Mile Run Test, or the Three-Minute Step Test—to find your recovery heart rate.

Cardiorespiratory: One-Mile Walk Test or 1.5-Mile Run Test

For this test, you can choose to walk or run to determine your current cardiorespiratory level.

- Purpose: This test estimates your level of cardiorespiratory fitness based on the time it takes you to walk exactly one mile or to run 1.5 miles as fast as you can.
- Equipment needed: Stopwatch.

- Plan a route: Choose a path near your home or use your local high school running track and measure one mile for the walk test or 1.5 miles if you are going to do the run test.

Directions:

- For these tests try to finish the test as quickly as possible without becoming too breathless.
- Aim to raise your heart rate above 120 beats per minute.
- Use a stopwatch to monitor time elapsed for testing results.
- Record your time in minutes and seconds in the space(s) provided below.

Timed Walk or Run Test

Men

Age	13-19 Walk	13-19 1.5 Mile Run	20-29 Walk	20-29 1.5 Mile Run	30-39 Walk	30-39 1.5 Mile Run
Excellent	11	<9:40	11:30	<10:45	12	<11:30
Good	11:01–12:45	9:41–10:48	11:31–13:15	10:46–12	12:01–13:30	11:31–13
Fair	12:46–14:10	10:49–12:10	13:16–14	12:01–14	13:31–15:15	13:01–15:35
Poor	14:11–15	12:11–15:30	14:01–15:30	14:01–16	15:16–17	15:36–17:30
Very poor	>15:01	>15:31	>15:31	>16:01	>17:01	>17:31

Women

Age	13-19 Walk	13-19 1.5 Mile Run	20-29 Walk	20-29 1.5 Mile Run	30-39 Walk	30-39 1.5 Mile Run
Excellent	<11:06	<12:29	<12	<13:30	<12:45	<14:30
Good	11:07–13	12:30–14:30	12:01–13:15	13:31–15:54	12:46–14	14:31–16:30
Fair	13:01–14:30	14:31–16:54	13:16–14:06	15:55–18:30	14:01–15:45	16:31–19
Poor	14:31–15:06	16:55–18:30	14:07–16	18:31–19	15:46–17	19:01–19:30
Very poor	>15:07	>18:31	>16:01	>19:01	>17:01	>19:31

*Add 1 second for to each category after age 39 for more accurate results on the 1-mile walk / run tests or log onto http://www.sxrx.net/Testing/YMCATesting.html and use the aerobic calculator.

One-Mile Walk: _____ Minutes _____ Seconds

1.5-Mile Run: _____ Minutes _____ Seconds

Cardiorespiratory:
Three-Minute Step Test

This simple three-minute test can provide you with a wealth of information about your cardiorespiratory condition before you officially start an exercise program.

- Purpose: This test estimates the level of your cardiorespiratory fitness.
- Equipment needed: Metronome (or you can pace yourself as described in the directions below), stopwatch, twelve-inch high step or sturdy box.
- Information: Using a metronome will help you stay on your target pace. Set the metronome for ninety-six beats a minute. If you do not have a metronome, the easiest way to maintain your pace is to make one full revolution of steps about every three seconds; therefore, stepping up/right foot, up/left foot, down/right foot, down/left foot should take approximately three seconds to complete to stay on target pace.

Directions:

- For this assessment, you will step up and down on a twelve-inch high box for three minutes and then wait one minute before taking your recovery pulse.
- Step up onto the center of the box with the

right foot, making sure that the heel makes contact first; then follow with the left foot.

- Once both feet are flat on the box, transfer your weight to your left foot and step down to the ground with your right foot, followed by the left.
- Movement will be this sequence: up (right foot), up (left foot), down (right foot), down (left foot).

After your three minutes of stepping, count your pulse beats for one full minute. Record your results in the space provided below.

3 Minute Step Test

Men

Age	18–25	26–35	36–45	46–55	56–65	65+
Excellent	<79	<81	<83	<87	<86	<88
Good	79–89	81–89	83–96	87–97	86–97	88–96
Above average	90–99	90–99	97–103	98–105	98–103	97–103
Average	100–105	100–107	104–112	106–116	104–112	104–113
Below average	106–116	108–117	113–119	116–122	113–120	114–120
Poor	117–128	118–128	120–130	123–132	121–129	121–130
Very poor	>128	>128	>130	>132	>129	>130

Women

Age	18–25	26–35	36–45	46–55	56–65	65+
Excellent	<85	<88	<90	<94	<95	<90
Good	85–98	88–99	90–102	94–104	95–104	90–102
Above average	99–108	100–111	103–110	105–115	105–112	103–115
Average	109–117	112–119	111–118	116–120	113–118	116–122
Below average	118–126	120–126	119–128	121–126	119–128	123–128
Poor	127–140	127–138	129–140	127–135	129–139	129–134
Very poor	>140	>138	>140	>135	>139	>134

_____ bpm

FLEXIBILITY TEST

Flexibility is important for the prevention of injury and joint wear and tear as you begin to consider adding more exercise into your daily routine. Many would-be fitness buffs get sidelined the first week they suit up because of lack of stretching, poor flexibility, and the injuries that can occur from this disastrous combination.

Poor flexibility of the lower back and hamstrings can lead to knee and back pain, bulging and herniated disks, along with cartilage breakdown in the knees and hips, and even joint replacement over time. The Sit and Reach Test below will test your flexibility so that you know where you stand—*before* you start to run.

Flexibility: Sit and Reach Test

To assess your flexibility of the lower back and hamstrings, we use the Sit and Reach Test found below.

- Purpose: To evaluate the flexibility of the lower back and hamstring muscles.
- Equipment needed: Yardstick or soft tape.

Directions:

- Remove your shoes and sit down.
- Take the yardstick or soft tape and place it flat on the floor with the fifteen-inch mark directly even with the heels of your feet. The one-inch mark will be closest to your body.
- Place your feet approximately twelve inches apart with your legs extended in front of you.

- Reaching forward with the fingertips on both hands even and palms facing down, try to touch the highest number you can possibly reach on the measuring device. Be sure to use slow, controlled movements and refrain from bouncing to ensure an accurate assessment, and from bending the knees, legs should remain completely straightened during the reaching phase.
- Use your best score out of three tries.
- Record the number of inches the tips of both hands reached evenly.

Sit & Reach Test

Men

Age	18–25	26–35	36–45	46–55	56–65	65+
Excellent	>20	>20	>19	>19	>17	>17
Good	19–20	18–19	17–19	16–18	16–17	13–15
Above average	17–18	16–17	15–17	14–15	12–14	11–13
Average	15–16	15	13–15	12–13	10–12	9–11
Below average	13–14	12–14	11–12	10–11	8–10	8–9
Poor	10–12	10–11	9–10	7–10	5–8	5–7
Very poor	<9	<10	<8	>7	<5	<5

Women

Age	18–25	26–35	36–45	46–55	56–65	65+
Excellent	>24	>23	>22	>21	>25	>25
Good	22–23	20–22	19–21	19–20	18–19	18–19
Above average	20–21	19–20	18	17–18	16–17	16–17
Average	18–19	18	16–17	15–16	15	14–15
Below average	16–17	16–17	14–15	14	13–14	12–13
Poor	14–15	14–15	11–13	11–13	10–12	10–11
Very poor	<13	<13	<10	<10	<10	<8

Flexibility: Sit and Reach Test _____

MUSCLE STRENGTH AND ENDURANCE TEST

Poor upper body strength and endurance can be an indicator of muscle imbalances, which, if left uncorrected over time, could lead to injury. It is important to assess the strength of your muscles and how much endurance you presently have before moving forward with your *Think Fit 2 Be Fit* program.

Muscle Strength: Push-Up Test

The one-minute Push-Up Test assesses your muscle strength, both of the upper body and core.

- Purpose: To evaluate the strength of the muscles located in the chest, triceps, bicep, shoulders, traps, and core.
- Equipment needed: None.

Directions:

- Lie flat on the floor face down with the palms of your hands placed near the shoulders and pressed flat on the floor.
- If necessary, you may do modified push-ups from your knees instead of your feet, but be sure to make a notation on your assessment sheet for future monitoring of strength improvements.
- Push your body up, while keeping your core tight for support, until your arms are fully extended. Your entire body should remain

straight and flat during the entire range of motion.

- Do as many push-ups as you can, using correct form, for one full minute.
- In the space provided below, record the number push-ups you completed in the allotted time.

Push-Up Test

Men

Age	17–19	20–29	30–39	40–49	50–59	60–65
Excellent	>51	>43	>37	>31	>28	>27
Good	35–50	30–42	25–36	21–30	18–27	17–26
Average	19–34	17–29	13–24	11–20	9–17	6–16
Below average	4–18	4–16	2–12	1–10	1–8	1–5
Poor	<3	<3	<1	0	0	0

Women

Age	17–19	20–29	30–39	40–49	50–59	60–65
Excellent	>32	>33	>34	>28	>23	>21
Good	21–32	23–32	22–33	18–27	15–22	13–20
Average	11–20	12–22	10–21	8–17	7–14	5–12
Below average	1–10	1–11	1–9	1–7	1–6	1–4
Poor	0	0	0	0	0	0

Muscle Strength: Push-Up Test _____

Muscle Endurance: Crunch Test

The one-minute Crunch Test assesses the endurance of your abdominal muscles.

- Purpose: To evaluate abdominal muscular strength and endurance.
- Equipment needed: None.

Directions:

- Lie on your back with your knees bent, feet flat on the floor, and heels should be between twelve and eighteen inches away from your buttocks.
- Do not hold your feet down with anything because this changes the muscles stressed in the test and will alter correct results.
- Place your hand behind your head, but only place your fingertips on your head so as to prevent pulling on the neck. Keep your elbows in line with your ears (pointing straight out to the sides) during the entire range of motion.
- Make sure that you move only your upper back and chest throughout this movement. The goal is to curl your chest into your belly button during the movement.
- Do as many curls as you can in one minute, using correct form.
- Record the number of curls completed in the space provided below.

1-Minute Crunch Test

Men

Age	<35	35 – 44	45+
Excellent	60	50	40
Good	45	40	25
Marginal	30	25	15
Needs work	10	15	5

Women

Age	<35	35 – 44	45+
Excellent	50	40	30
Good	40	25	15
Marginal	25	15	10
Needs work	10	6	4

Muscle Endurance: Crunch Test _____

BEFORE AND AFTER PICTURES

Have you ever looked at old pictures of yourself and thought, *Gosh, I didn't realize how skinny I was then,* or *Wow, I really ballooned up in weight during that time?* And yet, at that time, you never really realized what was happening?

Change is like that, particularly physical change. Yes, we all look in the mirror before work every day or check our makeup in the compact or glance at ourselves in a reflective window as we walk by, but such quick "snapshots" don't really tell the whole story.

Taking before and after pictures of yourself can be a great motivational tool for monitoring your progress throughout the *Think Fit 2 Be Fit* program and for motivating you to succeed each day. Even though you see yourself in the mirror every day, so many of the small changes you are making go unnoticed from week to week.

By taking pictures, you will be able see more noticeable changes in your body composition than you may have noticed in the mirror. Another common change that you may note is that your skin has a healthier tone to it or that your posture looks altogether better.

You can chart your progress multiple times over the course of this program, but for starters, here is a great place to paste your first "before" picture and, right next to it, an "after" picture later, when you feel you've really accomplished some significant change:

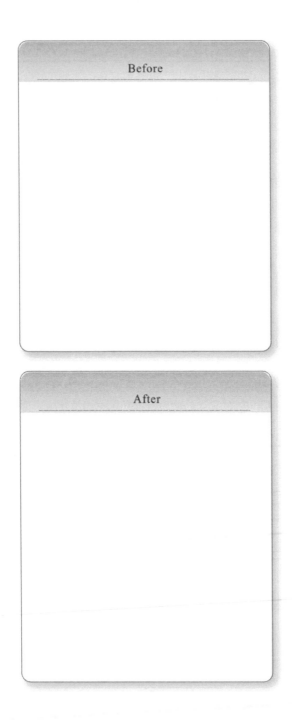

Before

After

TRACK YOUR RESULTS

Here is a handy chart you can use to write down the measurements provided in this section.

GENERAL	Date	Score	Date	Score	Date	Score	Date	Score	Goal
Age:									
Height:									
Weight:									
BMI:									
BODY COMPOSITION									
Body Fat:									
Fat Weight:									
Lean Weight:									
Waist to Hip Ratio:									
GIRTH MEASUREMENTS									
Shoulders:									
Chest:									
Upper Arm:									
Flexed Bicep:									
Forearm:									
Waist:									
Hips									
Upper Thigh									
Calf									
CARDIOVASCULAR FITNESS									
Avg RHR:									
Cardio Test:									
FLEXIBILITY									
Sit & Reach:									
STRENGTH & ENDURANCE TESTING									
Crunches:									
Push-ups									

Use these self-assessment results as a measurement of where you started. They can be great aids for determining where to set your bar of standards, when you're making results and when you're not, as well as a median of where you stand when compared to the rest of the population. The results are meant to be a motivational tool for getting started as well as staying motivated, especially when you assess periodically.

What makes us unique as individuals is our experience. Every experience creates an opportunity for personal growth. By learning this new information you'll add to your experiences of life, which will expand your mind in ways that can aid you in developing a fitness-focused lifestyle. The more you implement and practice these concepts and tips from this program, the greater the chance of you succeeding at reaching your personal wellness goals and beyond.

Just remember that it doesn't matter when you get there as long as you never stop thinking fit, because thinking it will manifest it. As the saying goes, "Rome wasn't built in a day." You didn't get out of shape in a day, so it won't take you a day to get back into shape. Just take things one day at a time, one change at a time, and you'll be fit faster than you ever imagined.

Bibliography

Albury, Christine. "Why Babies Need Full-Fat Foods American Chronicle | Why Babies Need Full-Fat Foods." American Chronicle   American Chronicle   . http://www.americanchronicle.com/articles/23601   (accessed June 7, 2008).

Bauer, Joy. "Raise a glass! Wine's health benefits—TODAY Health." Breaking News, Weather, Business, Health, Entertainment, Sports, Politics, Travel, Science, Technology, Local, US & World News—msnbc.com. http://www.msnbc.msn.com/id/21478144/   (accessed June 19, 2008).

"Carbohydrate   metabolism—Psychology   Wiki." Psychology   Wiki.   http://psychology.wikia.com/wiki/Carbohydrate_metabolism (accessed October 18, 2008).

Carmona, M.D., M.P.H., F.A.C.S., Richard H. "The Obesity Crisis in America." Office of the Surgeon General (OSG). http://www.surgeongeneral.gov/news/testimony/obesity07162003.htm   (accessed   September 16, 2005).

Carmona, M.D., M.P.H., F.A.C.S., Richard H. . "The Obesity Crisis in America." Office of the Surgeon General (OSG). http://www.surgeongeneral.gov/news/

testimony/obesity07162003.htm (accessed April 17, 2008).

Cromie, William J. "Harvard Gazette: Meditation changes temperatures." HPAC - Harvard Public Affairs & Communications. http://www.news.harvard.edu/gazette/2002/04.18/09-tummo.html (accessed February 16, 2007).

DeNoon, Daniel J. "Long-Distance Runners Risk Bone Loss." WebMD—Better information. Better health. http://www.webmd.com/osteoporosis/news/20030127/long-distance-runners-risk-bone-loss (accessed February 15, 2007).

ACE. "Fit Facts." Fit Facts from The American Council on Exercise. www.nmcphc.med.navy.mil/downloads/healthyliv/physfit/Newsletters/ACE/General_Exercise/Periodized_Training_Why_Its_Important.pdf (accessed July 19, 2008).

Freudenrich Ph.D., Craig. "Howstuffworks "How Alcohol Works"." TLC Cooking "Food and Recipes". http://recipes.howstuffworks.com/alcohol.htm/printable (accessed May 2, 2009).

Goleman, Daniel. "Probing the Enigma of Multiple Personality—NYTimes.com." The New York Times—Breaking News, World News & Multimedia. http://www.nytimes.com/1988/06/28/science/probing-the-enigma-of-multiple-personality.html?pagewanted=1 (accessed July 10, 2007).

American Heart Association. "Go Red For Women: Press Release." Go Red For Women. http://www.goredforwomen.org/press_release.aspx?release_id=926 (accessed August 1, 2010).

Higdon, Ph.D., Jane. "Linus Pauling Institute at Oregon State University." Linus Pauling Institute at Oregon State University. http://lpi.oregonstate.edu/infocenter/phytochemicals/resveratrol/ (accessed May 16, 2009).

Johnson, Brandon. "USDA Sodium Recommendations—What Are They and Why Should You Care?" EzineArticles Submission—Submit Your Best Quality Original Articles For Massive Exposure, Ezine Publishers Get 25 Free Article Reprints. http://ezinearticles.com/?USDA-Sodium-Recommendations---What-Are-They-and-Why-Should-You-Care?&id=2121366 (accessed August 2, 2010).

Jones, Jeffrey M. "In U.S., More Would Like to Lose Weight Than Are Trying To." Gallup.Com—Daily News, Polls, Public Opinion on Government, Politics, Economics, Management. http://www.gallup.com/poll/124448/in-u.s.-more-lose-weight-than-trying-to.aspx (accessed February 16, 2010).

Katch, Frank I., and William D. McArdle. *2.F r a n k I. Katch and William D. McArdle â€œIntroudction to Nutrition, Exercise and Health.* 1988. Reprint, Amherst: Fitness Technologies, 1993.

Lemon, PhD, Peter W.R. . "Beyond the Zone: Protein Needs of Active Individuals." Journal Of American College of Nutrition. www.jacn.org/cgi/content/full/19/suppl_5/513S (accessed May 25, 2009).

Encarta & MSN. "MSN Encarta." MSN Encarta. encarta.msn.com/encnet/features/dictionary/dictionary-home.aspx (accessed May 20, 2007).

Macpherson, Gordon. *Black's Medical Dictionary, 39th Edition (Black's Medical Dictionary)*. 39th ed. Lanham, Maryland: Madison Books, 1999.

Minkel, JR. "Supersize Me-and All My Friends." Medical News Today: Health News. http://www.medicalnewstoday.com/articles/78071.php (accessed May 19, 2009).

USDA. "MyPyramid.gov." MyPyramid.gov. http://www.mypyramid.gov/ (accessed May 17, 2005).

Center for Disease Control. "National Diabetes Fact Sheet, 2007." http://www.searchfordiabetes.org. www.searchfordiabetes.org/public/documents/CDCFact2008.pdf (accessed July 20, 2008).

Nippoldt, M.D., Todd B. "Salt craving: A symptom of Addison's disease?—MayoClinic.com." Mayo Clinic medical information and tools for healthy living—MayoClinic.com. http://www.mayoclinic.com/health/salt-craving/AN01597 (accessed October 16, 2008).

http://www.cnpp.usda.gov. "Nutrient Content." Nutrient Content. www.cnpp.usda.gov/publications/foodsupply/FoodSupply1909–2000.pdf (accessed December 19, 2006).

O'Riordan, Michael. "theheart.org: Cardiology news, educational programming, and opinions." theheart.org: Cardiology news, educational programming, and opinions. http://www.theheart.org/article/1039173.do (accessed January 13, 2010).

"Pancreas Transplantation." Bing. https://ssl.search. live.com/health/article.aspx?id=articles%2fmlp%2fpage s%2f1%2fPancreas_Transplantation.htm&qu=Pancreas (accessed October 25, 2009).

Peale, Norman Vincent. *The Power of Positive Thinking.* New Ed ed.: Vermilion, 1990.

Science News Magazine of the Society and the Public. "Protein links metabolism and circadian rhythms." Science News. hoodcenter.dartmouth.edu/publications/ documents/TheACTIIStudy_http://www.sciencenews. org/view/generic/id/34438/title/Protein_links_metabo-lism_and_circadian_rhythms.pdf (accessed October 20, 2008).

Robbins, Anthony. *Anthony Robbins Get The Edge: Transcript—A 7 Day Program to Transform Your Life & Personal Journal.* San Diego: Robbins Research International, 2002.

Siebert, Richard J. *American Council on Exercise Personal Trainer Manual.* 1991. Reprint, San Diego: Amer Council On Exercise, 1991.

Stanley, Thomas J. *The Millionaire Mind.* Kansas City: Andrews McMeel Publishing, 2001.

Super Size Me. DVD. Directed by Morgan Spurlock. Manhattan: Hart Sharp Video, 2004.

Sylver, Marshall. *Passion Profit and Power.* New York: Simon, 1995.

"The Affects of Caffeine on Weight Loss." Teeccino CaffÃ©. www.teeccino.com/weightloss.aspx (accessed October 25, 2009).

What the Bleep Do We Know!?. DVD. Directed by William Arntz. Tucson: 20th Century Fox, 2004.

YMCA. "YMCA Fitness Assessment." ExRx (Exercise Prescription) on the Net. http://www.exrx.net/Testing/YMCATesting.html (accessed May 24, 2009).

"carbohydrate (biochemistry)—Britannica Online Encyclopedia." Encyclopedia—Britannica Online Encyclopedia. http://www.britannica.com/EBchecked/topic/94687/carbohydrate (accessed October 5, 2008).

Photos of Tammy

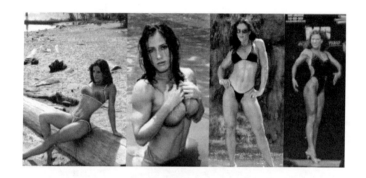

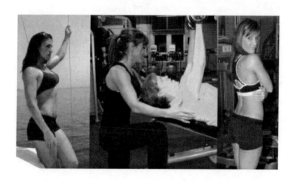

Tammy Polenz
Vedas
1360 E. 9th St., Suite 640
Cleveland, OH 44114
www.vedasfitness.com
Office: 216.298.5115